THIS JOURNAL BELONGS TO:

_____

THE skinnytaste™
MEAL PLANNER

REVISED EDITION

GINA HOMOLKA

CLARKSON POTTER/PUBLISHERS
NEW YORK

So many Skinnytaste fans use this meal planner every week, and based on your feedback, and my personal experience meal planning each week, I made some improvements so this journal is better than ever. With a new design and format, we now have more space to meal plan, a weekly shopping list, a notes column for extra reminders, boxes to check off your goals each day, and a spiral binding so the pages stay open for easier writing.

When I started trying to lose weight a few years ago, I found that the two things that made the biggest difference were cooking fresh, from-scratch, healthy dinners at home, where I was in control of what went into my meals, and tracking everything I ate so I knew exactly what (and how much) I was eating. Cooking greatly improved the quality and taste of my meals, and tracking helped clue me in to what foods to eat, what foods to limit, and how to make healthier daily choices.

So many readers of my blog, Skinnytaste.com, and my cookbooks, *The Skinnytaste Cookbook* and *Skinnytaste Fast and Slow*, are smart, proactive people who are ready to make a change in the name of health. That's why they like my recipes, which are not only full-flavored, but also surprisingly low in fat and calories—so you don't feel like you're eating diet food or missing out on the good stuff. After all, if you don't enjoy the process, it isn't likely to become a lifelong habit! With these types of folks in mind, I've created *The Skinnytaste Meal Planner.*

This journal is a daily tool to help you plan your meals and track your eating, as well as schedule your exercise activities, throughout the week. In the Weekly Meal Planner pages, you have a bird's-eye view of the week; this is where you can decide what days you have time to cook, which days will be leftover dinners, and how to otherwise organize your approach to cooking for the week.

On the Calories/Points Tracker pages, there's space to write down all the foods you eat each day, along with a place to log the amount of calories or points consumed. That way, you can see just how much is coming in—and you'll see if one particular meal or snack is throwing you off your goal! The last page of each week includes a box for tracking your exercise, since being active and burning calories day by day is also essential to being healthy.

Throughout the journal I've included motivational quotes, which get me going on days when I really need it. An inspirational phrase can instantly fill me with optimism and help me make good on my promises to myself! There are also notes on everyday superfoods—certain ingredients that are nutritional powerhouses—as well as twenty recipes.

Taking charge of your cooking and eating habits can make a big impact on your health and weight. I hope that *The Skinnytaste Meal Planner* is a helpful tool for you to get on the road to your very best self—and have fun while you're at it!

I truly believe that the best way to achieve your goals is to hold yourself accountable along the way. And diet and exercise are no exception!

When I began my journey years ago, I was shocked by what I learned when I actually wrote down what I ate in a day. I'd always thought I ate lean and light, and that I was fairly active. But I realized that every day I was inadvertently sneaking in bites of food that added up fast, and that my "exercise" didn't actually burn any calories of note. Seeing the real deal on paper made me snap to it! I finally knew where I was slipping up and why I wasn't seeing results—then I was able to determine how to get things under control.

The two sections of this journal are meant to work in tandem.

Weekly Meal Planner

At the beginning of the week, state what your goal (or goals) for that week is (are)—what do you want to try to do, more or less, during that week? Do you want to try a new food, or go cold turkey on sugar-packed sodas? Maybe you want to try swapping in almond milk for full-fat cow's milk, or be more diligent in packing healthy snacks to take to work so that you don't visit the vending machine every afternoon. Be creative in this section and think of things that challenge you to be mindful whenever you eat. And you can even write exercise goals here, too! Do you want to try a spin class for the first time, or walk with a friend three mornings a week? Write it down. At the end of the week, you can review your goals and see if you followed through—or decide if you should carry a goal into the next week.

Next, plan your meals for the week with your goal or goals in mind. You'll notice that there are spaces grouped with the letters B, L, and D. Those stand for

Breakfast, Lunch, and Dinner. No matter how much any of us loves to cook, it still takes a good amount of planning and preparing to pull off! With busy schedules and the rigors of grocery shopping, being proactive will help you succeed. When I was losing weight, I found that I ate healthier foods when I was in control of the dishes—and that meant cooking. Aim for a certain number of days to cook each week, and write out which days those will be. Then you'll be better able to arrange other things in your week so that you also have time to cook. Also, come up with some ideas for your leftovers! I love it when I make a little extra of a dish so that I can enjoy it again later in the week—either just as they are, or remade into another delicious dish. Leftovers are great to pack for work, too.

Calories/Points and Exercise Tracker

After planning, it's time to be accountable! And that's where the tracker pages come into the picture. As I said before, it's one thing to think you eat healthfully, but it's another thing to know for sure. Use these pages to write down every single thing you eat in a day. Did you skip breakfast? Okay, but don't do that again (breakfast is important!). A colleague brought in cookies and you had half of one? Write it down! You'll be surprised to see how many little things like these accumulate. In the space next to where you wrote down each dish or item of food consumed, add the calories of those foods. This is where your eyes may be opened! Sometimes a seemingly innocent sandwich from your local shop is a calorie bomb in disguise. And sometimes you'll find that your salad is healthier than you thought! It'll probably go both ways, and by tracking these calorie counts, you'll begin to find a way to better tailor your eating so that you stay fit and only indulge in comfort foods every now and again.

Don't forget to exercise! Moving your body is just as pivotal to overall health as eating well is, so don't neglect this side of the equation. Aim for at least 20 minutes of exercise most days of the week—and work your way up to more! Have fun with it. Join a running group so your exercise time is social, or find a fun class at your gym to keep you motivated. Craft a new playlist to keep your energy high, and get a couple of new tank tops (hey, looking good can help you feel good!). There are so many ways to accumulate data on how many calories you burned by performing various activities, from the counters on gym machines to those handy personal trackers like FitBit. You can also go online to MyFitnessPal.com/exercise/lookup for information on calories burned that takes into account your weight.

Above all, I hope that this journal is helpful to you. Feeling confident in yourself, being active and fit, and knowing that you're fueling your body with the best foods possible will boost your happiness. And accomplishing your goals will give you a surge of joy that will spread throughout your life! Check out my examples of how to fill in this journal on pages 12–17, following the "11 Easy Ways" section.

Getting Started

It can be difficult to take those first steps toward a healthier lifestyle—I've been there and know firsthand! But all you need to do is start simple: learn what foods are truly good for you and how many calories you need per day, and then work in changes to your eating and exercise week by week.

So, how do you know how many calories you're supposed to aim for each day? This is a good first question to answer, since that number will be your main guide to shedding weight. If you're following a points-based plan, then you know how important calories are, and you're likely familiar with how many you should be consuming. A basic rule of thumb is that an average adult woman should consume 1,500 to 1,600 calories per day in order to see a healthy weight loss of approximately two pounds per week. Bear in mind, though, that many factors, such as height, weight, and activity level, greatly influence this number. There are great calorie calculators online; I recommend checking out www.mayoclinic .org/calorie-calculator/itt-20084939 to find the right daily caloric intake for you.

11 EASY WAYS TO EAT CLEAN

Health before weight loss is my first priority, so eating clean is always my main focus. And by cleaning your diet and focusing on foods that make your calories count, the pounds will naturally come off. Work on eating the healthiest options in each food group (fresh fruits and vegetables, lean protein, good fats, and whole grains) while eliminating from your diet the not-so-healthy ones (processed foods, refined grains, refined sugars, and unhealthy fats). Here are a few simple tips to get you started and reprogram your eating habits.

1. Read Your Labels

The first step to cleaning up your diet is to limit or avoid the amount of processed or refined food you consume. This is easier than you think. Look at the ingredient list on the back of the packaged foods before you purchase them. If there's a long list of ingredients (more than five), or if there are ingredients you can't pronounce, stay away. If you're unsure the next time you're in the supermarket, I highly recommend the smartphone app called Fooducate, which lets you scan the items in the supermarket, and then the app grades the food, explains the ingredients listed, and suggests healthier alternatives.

2. Homemade Is Healthier

Although it takes a little more time, cooking your favorite foods—such as macaroni and cheese, marinara sauce, bread crumbs, granola bars, and baked goods—rather than buying them from a box or the frozen aisle will not only be cleaner and healthier, they'll taste better, too. Again, check the label to see how many unnatural foods are hiding in that frozen apple pie!

3. Drink More Water

Our bodies need water for everything! Drinking enough water is key to feeling great. And did you know that sometimes thirst can be mistaken for hunger? Make sure you don't reach for a snack when what you really need is a glass of water! Your goal should be to drink approximately 2 liters a day. If you're in the habit of drinking soda, try switching to seltzer that you flavor with fresh-squeezed citrus or fresh mint.

4. Eat More Veggies

On average, as a nation, we are still behind the daily recommended intake of vegetables, which is 2½ to 3 cups for adults. Make it a goal to increase your veggie consumption, and you'll be adding healthful vitamins, minerals, and fiber every day. And try going meatless once a week! Meatless Mondays are a great way to focus on veggie meals and can make it fun for your family, too.

5. Choose Organic When Possible

Nowadays, organic fruits and vegetables are widely available. Most grocery stores, and even Walmart, stock lots of clean produce. The more organic foods you eat, the less you fill your body with harmful chemicals. If it's not in your budget to eat everything organic, at least try to avoid the Environmental Working Group's Dirty Dozen: apples, celery, cherries, grapes, nectarines, peaches, pears, potatoes, spinach, strawberries, sweet bell peppers, and tomatoes.

6. Choose Lean Protein

Nothing will keep you feeling full like protein! It's necessary for muscle growth, too, and is a must every day. Focus on eating lean proteins so that you keep calories low while getting the good stuff. Lean proteins include: chicken breast, eggs, legumes, tofu, edamame, turkey, roast beef, pork tenderloin, Greek yogurt, low-fat milk, cottage cheese, nuts and nut butters, seeds, and fish.

7. Opt for Whole Grains

We are so lucky these days that grocery stores stock a wide variety of excellent whole grains, which are leaps and bounds more healthy than their processed counterparts. Reach for oatmeal and brown rice, whole wheat bread, granola, quinoa, barley, farro, bulgur, spelt, and more.

8. Snack on More Fruit

So many foods advertised today as "snacks" have us reaching for crackers, chips, cookies, and other carbs—many of which are loaded with salt and refined sugars. Reach instead for fresh fruits, which have natural sugars, as well as lots of vitamins, minerals, and fiber. Pack them in your bag so that you're always armed when hunger strikes!

9. Consume Healthy Fats

Not all fat is bad for you! That's a myth of the past, but now we know that many healthy fats are excellent parts of a good diet. Some foods with good fats to work into your weekly eating are olives, salmon, avocados, nuts, nut butter, pumpkin seeds, sesame seeds, and olive oil.

10. Cut Back on Sugar

It is amazing the things that are packed with sugar these days! Sugar is almost a way of life for Americans, but thankfully the word is out that too much in your diet can harm your health in many ways—and lots of people are learning to make better choices. Aim to decrease the sugar you consume a little every day. A great place to start is by eliminating soda. You'll avoid about 44 grams of sugar per can of cola!

11. Limit Your Cocktails

I love a good cocktail or glass of wine at the end of the day, and especially when out with girlfriends! But I also know that drinks can be extremely high in calories—more than 200 calories for one drink! Even a glass of red wine has about 125. The caloric impact of cocktails adds up fast, so aim to limit your consumption and avoid sugary drinks.

Weekly Meal Planner

DATE _5 / 1 / 17_ TO _5 / 7 / 17_

1. Workout 4 days

M T W T F S S
☒ ☐ ☒ ☒ ☐ ☐ ☒

2. Drink 8-10 cups of water a day

M T W T F S S
☒ ☒ ☒ ☒ ☒ ☒ ☒

3. Try a new gym class!

M T W T F S S
☐ ☐ ☒ ☐ ☐ ☐ ☐

	MONDAY
B	Eggs, toast, banana
L	Greek Salad with Grilled Chicken
D	Grilled Lamb Chops with Mint Yogurt Sauce
	Quinoa Tabbouleh
	TUESDAY
B	Smoothie
L	Leftover Quinoa Tabbouleh
D	Skinny Broccoli Mac and Cheese
	House Salad Made with Love
	WEDNESDAY
B	Yogurt, coffee
L	Egg, tomato, and scallion sandwich
D	Coconut Chicken Salad
	Piña Colada Chia Pudding
	THURSDAY
B	Overnight oats, coffee
L	Tuna avocado sandwich
D	Skinny Chicken Parmesan
	Lemon Roasted Asparagus
	FRIDAY
B	Eggs, toast, banana
L	Leftovers
D	Pizza night! Order from Nick's

SHOPPING LIST

- [ ] milk
- [ ] strawberries
- [ ] avocados
- [ ] eggs
- [ ]
- [ ]
- [ ]
- [ ]
- [ ]
- [ ]
- [ ]
- [ ]
- [ ]
- [ ]
- [ ]
- [ ]
- [ ]
- [ ]
- [ ]

> "Believe you can and
> you're halfway there."
>
> THEODORE ROOSEVELT

NOTES

SATURDAY	
B	Yogurt, coffee
L	Avocado toast with crab
D	So-Addicted Chicken Enchiladas with brown rice

SUNDAY	
B	Chocolate Chip Pancakes
L	Leftover enchilada, salad
D	Slow Cooker Picadillo with brown rice
	Summer Berry Cobbler

Calories/Points Tracker

DATE _5 / 1 / 17_ TO _5 / 7 / 17_

MONDAY			TUESDAY	
FOODS	Calories/Points		FOODS	Calories/Points
BREAKFAST				
Coffee with 1 tsp sugar 18			Coffee with 1 tsp sugar 18	
1 oz milk	18		1 oz milk	18
2 eggs	166		Green Monster	
1 ww toast	80		smoothie	254
Banana	105			
LUNCH				
Greek salad	300		Leftover quinoa	
3 oz grilled chicken	154		tabbouleh	110
			Pita	160
			Apple	91
DINNER				
Lamb chops	248		Broccoli mac	
Quinoa tabbouleh	154		and cheese	321
			House salad	117
SNACKS				
1 oz cheddar	114		1 cup cherries	87
1 oz cashews	162		1 oz pistachios	160
Peach	59		1 oz chocolate	149
DAILY TOTAL	1,578		DAILY TOTAL	1,485

WEDNESDAY		THURSDAY	
FOODS	Calories/ Points	FOODS	Calories/ Points
8 oz 0% Greek		PB&J overnight	
yogurt	130	oats	288
1 tbsp honey	64	2 coffees with	
½ oz walnuts	93	2 tsp sugar	32
Coffee with 1 tsp sugar	18	2 oz milk	32
1 oz milk	18		
Egg, tomato, scallion		2 oz ww bread w/ 2 oz	
sandwich	220	canned tuna,	
		¼ avocado, tomato,	
		and sprouts	300
		Peach	59
Coconut chicken		Chicken Parmesan	174
salad	340	2 oz pasta	200
6 oz white wine	142	Lemon asparagus	
Banana	105	(2 servings)	48
		6 oz white wine	142
Piña colada		Banana	105
chia pudding	161	5 oz yogurt	87
Chai tea latte	240	1 tbsp jam	10
DAILY TOTAL	1,531	DAILY TOTAL	1,477

Calories/Points Tracker

	FRIDAY			SATURDAY	
	FOODS	Calories/Points		FOODS	Calories/Points
BREAKFAST	Coffee with 1 tsp sugar	18		8 oz 0% Greek	
	1 oz milk	18		yogurt	130
	2 eggs	166		1 tbsp honey	64
	1 ww toast	80		½ oz walnuts	93
	Banana	105		Coffee with 1 tsp sugar	18
				1 oz milk	18
LUNCH	Chicken Parm	174		Avocado toast	
	Asparagus	48		with crab	484
				(2 pieces)	
DINNER	1 slice pizza	277		Chicken enhiladas	193
	Side salad	250		¾ cup brown rice	161
	5 oz wine	123		5 oz wine	123
SNACKS	Strawberries	49		Apple	95
	1 oz cheddar	114		1 oz cheddar	114
	DAILY TOTAL	1,422		DAILY TOTAL	1,493

WEEKLY EXERCISE TRACKER

SUNDAY	
FOODS	Calories/Points
Chocolate chip pancakes (2)	192
Coffee with 1 tsp sugar	18
1 oz milk	18
Leftover enchilada	194
Salad	200
Picadillo	207
3/4 cup brown rice	161
Summer berry cobbler	223
1 oz walnuts	185
Banana	105
DAILY TOTAL	1,503

ACTIVITY		
MON – walk 2 miles (4 mph)		
DISTANCE/DURATION/INTENSITY		CALORIES BURNED
30 minutes		170
WEDS – yoga		
1 hour		170
THURS – circuit training		
30 minutes		272
SUN – circuit training		
30 minutes		272
TOTAL CALORIES BURNED		884

MONDAY	1,578	- 170	=	1,408
TUESDAY	1,485	- 0	=	1,485
WEDNESDAY	1,531	- 170	=	1,361
THURSDAY	1,477	- 272	=	1,205
FRIDAY	1,422	- 0	=	1,422
SATURDAY	1,493	- 0	=	1,493
SUNDAY	1,503	- 272	=	1,231
WEEKLY CALORIES TOTALS	10,489	- 884	=	9,605
	Food	Exercise		Total

HEALTHY AND DELICIOUS INGREDIENTS SWAPS

One of my best Skinnytaste tricks is to swap out full-fat ingredients or those with empty calories for more nutritious items. You still get amazing flavor, with the bonus of better-for-you food! Here's a list of my favorite swaps to help you learn how to take your favorite recipes from diet saboteur to skinny.

↻ SWAP
Mashed avocado for mayo

Move over, mayo. Not only does avocado deliver monounsaturated fat, which helps protect the heart, and vitamin E, which is vital to immune function, but it also has nearly half the calories and fat of mayo. A 2-tablespoon serving of mayo has around 200 calories and 20 grams of fat, while that of a mashed avocado has only around 120 calories and 10 grams of fat.

↻ SWAP
Greek yogurt for mayo

Save calories and fat without sacrificing flavor. Greek yogurt has the same creamy consistency of mayo, but it offers some protein, which is more satiating than fat and carbs. Add a bit of red wine vinegar, and use it in place of mayo in mayonnaise-based salads. Or make a more conservative change: Swap out half the mayo for yogurt—you won't notice the difference.

↻ SWAP
Egg whites for whole eggs

When I make a dish that requires eggs, such as egg salad or omelets, I replace half of the whole eggs with egg whites. This allows me to cut back on cholesterol while still getting a healthy helping of satiating protein. I don't go totally yolk-free though, because there are some healthful nutrients (like the antioxidants lutein and zeaxanthin and the B vitamin choline) in the yolk.

↻ SWAP
Lettuce leaves for wraps or tortillas

Using fresh lettuce in place of wraps or tortillas is an easy way to cut your carb intake and increase the nutritional value of your meal. My favorite lettuce to use for this purpose is iceberg lettuce because the outer leaves are large and the texture is crisp. You can also try using romaine, Boston, or even cabbage.

⟳ SWAP
Mashed cauliflower for mashed potatoes

Steamed and mashed cauliflower has a very similar texture to mashed potatoes. But cauliflower is, well, a head above the potato because it's lower in calories and it may help protect against heart disease and cancer.

⟳ SWAP
Zucchini "noodles" for pasta

I use a spiralizer or a mandoline fitted with a julienne blade to cut zucchini into spaghetti-like strands. You can also use a potato peeler to cut them into ribbons (just make sure you leave out the "seedy" part in the middle or they end up too mushy). You can eat the strands raw, but I like to season them with salt and pepper and sauté them in a little oil for about 2 minutes. A good rule of thumb is to make one medium 8-ounce zucchini per person because it shrinks a little when it cooks.

⟳ SWAP
Spaghetti squash for pasta

Talk about a calorie savings: One cup of pasta has 220 calories, whereas a cup of spaghetti squash has only 42 calories. Plus, that cup of spaghetti squash is much more nutrient-dense, meaning it contains a lot more vitamins and minerals. Roast or microwave the squash, and then use a fork to pull apart and separate the spaghetti-like strands. The result: a slimmer, healthier alternative to pasta in the fall and winter months.

⟳ SWAP
Ground turkey or chicken for ground beef

There are times when I still prefer to cook with lean ground beef, but most of the time I replace the beef with ground turkey or chicken to cut back on saturated fat. It works for meat loaf, meatballs, chili, burgers, and more.

⟳ SWAP
Brown rice for white rice

To produce white rice (which keeps longer than brown rice), manu-facturers strip the kernel of its outer layer, also known as the bran. Unfortunately, that's where you'll find many of the good-for-you nutrients, including fiber and B vitamins. Stick with brown rice for the extra fiber and vitamins. Dried brown rice takes a little longer to cook than white; if you're short on time, buy parboiled brown rice, which is ready in about 10 minutes.

⟳ SWAP
Whole-grain bread for white bread

Replacing processed white bread with whole-grain bread is a simple way to get more vitamins, fiber, and vital nutrients. Although food producers try to add these health-promoting nutrients back to the product after processing, these unnatural sources are not as easily absorbed and digested by the body.

⟲ SWAP
Whole-grain pasta for white pasta

Whole-grain pasta has come a long way over the years. I find the flavor to be richer than white pasta, and it's certainly healthier—you'll get more fiber and vitamins by opting for whole grain. Nowadays, there are more choices than ever, including whole wheat pasta, brown rice pasta, and quinoa pasta, to name just a few.

⟲ SWAP
Oil mister for oil direct from a bottle

Oil helps add flavor and keeps food from sticking during the cooking process, but it's loaded with fat and calories. What's a chef to do? Try misting instead of pouring. I use at least three oil misters—one for olive oil, one for canola oil, and one for sesame oil. Remember, a little goes a long way.

⟲ SWAP
Oven frying for deep frying

You can achieve the same crispy golden texture you get from frying right in your own oven. It's easier and quicker, and (bonus!) there's no greasy mess to clean up.

⟲ SWAP
Avocado puree for butter

Avocado, which is creamy and nearly flavorless, can be used as a healthier stand-in for butter in cookies, cakes, and brownies. Avocados are loaded with vitamin E and heart-protecting monounsaturated fat, so you can feel a little less guilty about enjoying your splurge. You can generally swap equal amounts of well-mashed avocado for butter.

⟲ SWAP
Unsweetened applesauce for oil or butter

Applesauce is another great substitution for butter when making muffins, quick breads, and even pancakes. Plus, it adds some natural sweetness, so you can cut back on the sugar. **NOTE:** *Because applesauce doesn't contain fat, you still have to keep some of the butter or oil. It takes some experimenting to figure out how much to cut out. If you're making a favorite indulgent recipe, try swapping half the fat for applesauce the first time you make it, and then adjust accordingly the next time.*

⟳ SWAP
Ripe mashed bananas for oil or butter

Like avocados and applesauce, bananas have a creamy consistency that makes them an ideal replacement for fats in muffins, quick breads, and pancakes. They also add moisture and sweetness, so you can use less sugar. Another benefit: You'll get some potassium, fiber, and a handful of vitamins. Start by replacing half the fat with mashed bananas, and then adjust accordingly the next time.

⟳ SWAP
Prune puree for butter

Puree ½ cup of pitted prunes with ¼ cup of water in a blender or processor until smooth. The dark color and strong flavor of this fat substitute make it best suited for chocolate-based or heavily spiced baked goods, such as cookies, muffins, and quick breads. To replace 1 stick (½ cup) of butter, use ⅓ cup of prune puree.

⟳ SWAP
Stevia for sugar

Stevia, a zero-calorie sweetener, is up to 300 times sweeter than sugar. I usually use only a few drops of liquid stevia in place of sugar in smoothies. If you overdo it, the taste becomes bitter, so start with a little and taste as you go.

⟳ SWAP
Dates for sugar

Although dates are high in natural sugar, they're considered a low-glycemic-index food, meaning they won't spike your blood sugar. Medjool dates are my favorite because they're moist. Look for dates that are plump and free of crystallized sugar on the skins. To cook with them, soak them in hot water, and then remove the pits. Puree to use in smoothies, muffins, quick breads, pie fillings, or salad dressings.

⟳ SWAP
Fat-free frozen yogurt for ice cream

When I want to enjoy a dessert à la mode or whip up a low-fat milk shake, I always opt for fat-free frozen yogurt. Look for brands that have live active cultures for an extra health boost (these beneficial bacteria have been shown to improve digestive health).

EVERYDAY SUPERFOODS

A superfood is one that's loaded with nutrition and significantly helps boost your health in some way. Although these foods offer big benefits, they don't cost big bucks. Plus, they're easy to find—many of these health-promoting picks are available at your local grocery store or farmer's market—and incorporate into your diet. Here is a list of some of my favorite superfoods and information on how they keep you healthy from my friend and nutritionist Heather K. Jones; keep a lookout throughout the journal for superfood tips that use them:

❶ Blueberries

They may be small, but blueberries are nutritional powerhouses, packed with compounds that can help protect your heart, brain, eyes, and more. Blueberries contain polyphenols, which have antioxidant and anti-inflammatory properties that can ward off diseases like diabetes, cancer, and heart disease.

❷ Kiwifruit

One fuzzy fruit will nearly cover your daily vitamin C needs, is a great source of potassium, and is loaded with other good-for-you nutrients including folate, magnesium, and the phytochemical lutein, which helps protect your eyes. One study even found that the compounds in kiwifruit may help improve sleep.

❸ Oranges

This citrus fruit offers 3 grams of filling fiber, nearly all the vitamin C you need in a day, some vitamin A, and folate. In a study from researchers in the United Kingdom, women who ate the most citrus fruits, which are rich in the antioxidant flavanones, had a lower risk for stroke than women who consumed the least.

❹ Mushrooms

Loaded with fiber, selenium, B vitamins, and potassium, mushrooms have been shown to help protect against cancer. They can also be a good source of vitamin D, which promotes bone health and may play a role in the prevention of a variety of diseases, including heart disease. And with so many varieties to choose from—portobello, shiitake, morel, or white button, to name just a few—you're sure to find one that works in your favorite dishes.

❺ Cherries

Sure, cherries help make a mean pie, but they're so much more than simply pie filler. The little red orbs contain melatonin, the hormone that helps with sleep and may protect against some diseases. And their antioxidant and anti-inflammatory powers, courtesy of the fruits' anthocyanins, rival some of our best medicines—one study suggests cherries relieve pain better than aspirin.

6 Sweet potatoes

One sweet potato contains nearly 4 grams of fiber and covers your daily vitamin A requirements. It also chips in some vitamin C, potassium, iron, and magnesium. The orange spud is a super source of beta-carotene, an antioxidant that may reduce the risk for cancer. Another benefit of beta-carotene: It can protect your skin from aging and damage and give you a healthy glow.

7 Eggs

Eggs have gotten a bad rep over the years, but both egg whites and yolks contain healthful nutrients. The whites are a source of lean protein—there are 0 grams of saturated fat per 3-ounce serving. And the yolks are a rich source of the antioxidants lutein and zeaxanthin, both of which help protect the eyes. Although the yolks are high in dietary cholesterol, one study found that people who ate one egg a day for five weeks had higher antioxidant levels without seeing any increases in cholesterol.

8 Walnuts

On those days when you feel like a nut, it may be worth it to go for walnuts. In a study from the University of Pennsylvania, researchers found that walnuts had more (and higher quality) antioxidants than other nuts. Walnuts also contain the plant source of omega-3 fats called alpha-Linolenic acids (ALAs), which can help protect your heart, brain, and more.

9 Broccoli

A member of the cruciferous family like its cauliflower cousin, broccoli is a good source of fiber, calcium, folate, and vitamins A, C, and K. It's also packed with potent disease-fighting antioxidants, such as sulforaphane, kaempferol, quercetin, lutein, and zeaxanthin. Studies show that people who eat more broccoli have a lower risk for cancer.

10 Salmon

Need a reason to go fish? Here are some benefits to reeling in salmon: The fish is a source of lean protein and contains omega-3 fats, which prevent plaque formation in the arteries, reduce blood pressure, and decrease levels of triglycerides, a harmful fat found in the blood. For these reasons, the American Heart Association and other health groups recommend eating salmon and other fatty fish at least twice per week.

⑪ Yogurt

Yogurt can be a great source of protein, which is more satiating than fat and carbs. It's also loaded with calcium—an 8-ounce container covers nearly half of your daily needs for the bone-building mineral—and other vitamins and minerals. Some yogurt varieties earn extra points because they contain live active cultures of good bacteria, which have been shown to boost gut health. Be sure to steer clear of sweetened or flavored yogurts, which are more like desserts.

⑫ Kale

A good general nutrition guideline to keep in mind when produce shopping: The darker the color, the more antioxidants the fruit or vegetable usually contains. Perhaps that's why kale is so loaded with good-for-you compounds—including the phytochemicals lutein, zeaxanthin, beta-carotene, quercetin, and kaempferol—which have been shown to protect against cancer and other diseases. The dark leafy green also delivers a dose of vitamins A, C, and K, calcium and magnesium.

⑬ Apples

Apples have been shown to help reduce the risk for heart disease, cancer, asthma, and Alzheimer's. They may also help improve cognitive function, diabetes, weight control, and gut health. This may be because apples are rich in polyphenols, powerful antioxidants, and fiber, and also chip in some vitamin C and potassium. Enjoy them as a healthy snack, bake them into delicious desserts, have them as a savory side dish, or add them to your salad for a crunchy topping. How about them apples!

⑭ Flaxseeds

Flaxseeds are rich in fiber, ALAs (the plant form of omega-3 fatty acids), and lignans (plant compounds that act as antioxidants and phytoestrogens—a weaker form of the hormone estrogen—in the body). Research suggests that flaxseeds may help lower levels of A1C, a measure of blood sugar over three months, in people with diabetes. It may also reduce cholesterol in people with high cholesterol and help improve kidney function in people with lupus. In addition, flaxseeds seem to have some potential to fight prostate cancer.

⑮ Dark chocolate

Talk about sweet news—dark chocolate has been shown to protect the heart by lowering blood pressure, improving blood flow, and making platelets less sticky. Dark chocolate is made from cocoa, which contains flavonols, the same beneficial compounds found in grapes and wine. (Research suggests that dark chocolate has more antioxidants than milk or white chocolate.) Worried about your waistline? One study indicates that frequent chocolate eaters had a lower body mass index (a ratio of height to weight) than those who didn't enjoy chocolate regularly.

16 Green tea

It's tea time! Green tea is rich in antioxidants that may reduce your risk for diabetes, heart disease, and other conditions. One study found that those who drank six or more cups of green tea per day were 33 percent less likely to develop type 2 diabetes compared with those who drank less than one cup per day. Other research shows that people who drank green tea regularly for 10 years had less body fat and a smaller waist circumference than those who didn't. You can opt for regular green tea leaves or bags, or try the powdered form, called Matcha, to brew your own cup.

17 Garlic

This odorous vegetable may help with a number of conditions: Studies suggest that garlic may help reduce blood pressure by up to 8 percent in people with high blood pressure. It may also help keep arteries healthy and protect against a variety of cancers, including those of the colon, stomach, and rectum. The chemical that gives garlic its smell—allicin—also seems to be responsible for many of these health benefits.

18 Olive oil

Not all fats are created equal—there are good fats and then there are bad fats. Olive oil, without question, is a good fat. The oil, which is high in monounsaturated fat, the type that's heart-healthy, is a staple of the Mediterranean Diet, the eating style that is credited for the good health and longevity of the people living in that area. The benefits are numerous: Olive oil helps you feel full, protects against Alzheimer's, keeps your heart healthy, and boosts your brain power, to name just a few.

19 Avocados

Whether they're eaten plain, subbed for spreads like mayonnaise, mashed into guacamole, or used in a savory recipe, avocados are one of nature's finest—and most misunderstood—fruits. Historically slammed for their fat content, avocados are now lauded for their *beneficial* monounsaturated fats and omega-3s, which contribute to healthy cholesterol levels, prevent heart disease, and help us absorb the fat-soluble vitamins in the foods we pair with them. When selecting a ripe avocado, look for fruits that are firm and heavy and yield to gentle pressure without denting.

20 Tomatoes

No matter how you say it, tomatoes are nutrition superstars, thanks to their high content of lycopene, which has been shown to help protect against a variety of cancers, osteoporosis, heart disease, and more. And unlike other compounds, lycopene is more easily absorbed by the body when it's cooked, so tomato products like sauce may offer even more antioxidants than raw tomatoes.

FOOD & EXERCISE TRACKER

Track and plan your meals
and exercise goals for the week.

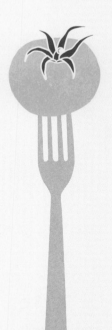

Weekly Meal Planner

DATE ___ / ___ / ___ TO ___ / ___ / ___

WEEKLY GOALS

1. _____
M T W T F S S
☐ ☐ ☐ ☐ ☐ ☐ ☐

2. _____
M T W T F S S
☐ ☐ ☐ ☐ ☐ ☐ ☐

3. _____
M T W T F S S
☐ ☐ ☐ ☐ ☐ ☐ ☐

MONDAY	
B	
L	
D	

TUESDAY	
B	
L	
D	

WEDNESDAY	
B	
L	
D	

THURSDAY	
B	
L	
D	

FRIDAY	
B	
L	
D	

SHOPPING LIST

- [ ] _____
- [ ] _____
- [ ] _____
- [ ] _____
- [ ] _____
- [ ] _____
- [ ] _____
- [ ] _____
- [ ] _____
- [ ] _____
- [ ] _____
- [ ] _____
- [ ] _____
- [ ] _____
- [ ] _____
- [ ] _____
- [ ] _____
- [ ] _____
- [ ] _____

> "Believe you can and
> you're halfway there."
>
> THEODORE ROOSEVELT

NOTES

_____

_____

_____

_____

_____

_____

_____

_____

_____

_____

_____

SATURDAY	
B	
L	
D	

SUNDAY	
B	
L	
D	

Calories/Points Tracker

DATE _____ / _____ / _____ TO _____ / _____ / _____

	MONDAY			TUESDAY	
	FOODS	Calories/Points		FOODS	Calories/Points
BREAKFAST					
LUNCH					
DINNER					
SNACKS					
	DAILY TOTAL			DAILY TOTAL	

WEDNESDAY		THURSDAY	
FOODS	Calories/Points	FOODS	Calories/Points
DAILY TOTAL		DAILY TOTAL	

Calories/Points Tracker

DATE ___ / ___ / ___ TO ___ / ___ / ___

	FRIDAY			SATURDAY	
	FOODS	Calories/Points		FOODS	Calories/Points
BREAKFAST					
LUNCH					
DINNER					
SNACKS					
	DAILY TOTAL			DAILY TOTAL	

WEEKLY EXERCISE TRACKER

ACTIVITY	
DISTANCE/DURATION/INTENSITY	CALORIES BURNED

SUNDAY	
FOODS	Calories/ Points
DAILY TOTAL	

TOTAL CALORIES BURNED	

MONDAY	-	=
TUESDAY	-	=
WEDNESDAY	-	=
THURSDAY	-	=
FRIDAY	-	=
SATURDAY	-	=
SUNDAY	-	=
WEEKLY CALORIES TOTALS	-	=
	Food	Exercise	Total

Weekly Meal Planner

WEEKLY GOALS

1. _____ M T W T F S S
   ☐ ☐ ☐ ☐ ☐ ☐ ☐

2. _____ M T W T F S S
   ☐ ☐ ☐ ☐ ☐ ☐ ☐

3. _____ M T W T F S S
   ☐ ☐ ☐ ☐ ☐ ☐ ☐

MONDAY
B
L
D

TUESDAY
B
L
D

WEDNESDAY
B
L
D

THURSDAY
B
L
D

FRIDAY
B
L
D

SHOPPING LIST

- [ ] _____
- [ ] _____
- [ ] _____
- [ ] _____
- [ ] _____
- [ ] _____
- [ ] _____
- [ ] _____
- [ ] _____
- [ ] _____
- [ ] _____
- [ ] _____
- [ ] _____
- [ ] _____
- [ ] _____
- [ ] _____
- [ ] _____
- [ ] _____

superfood BLUEBERRIES

Try tossing small but powerful blueberries in yogurt, cereal, or a smoothie, or just eat a handful on the go.

NOTES

_____
_____
_____
_____
_____
_____
_____
_____
_____
_____
_____
_____

SATURDAY	
B	
L	
D	

SUNDAY	
B	
L	
D	

Calories/Points Tracker

DATE ___/___/___ TO ___/___/___

	MONDAY			TUESDAY	
	FOODS	Calories/Points		FOODS	Calories/Points
BREAKFAST					
LUNCH					
DINNER					
SNACKS					
	DAILY TOTAL			DAILY TOTAL	

WEDNESDAY		THURSDAY	
FOODS	Calories/ Points	FOODS	Calories/ Points
DAILY TOTAL		DAILY TOTAL	

Calories/Points Tracker

DATE _____ / _____ / _____ TO _____ / _____ / _____

	FRIDAY			SATURDAY	
	FOODS	Calories/Points		FOODS	Calories/Points
BREAKFAST					
LUNCH					
DINNER					
SNACKS					
	DAILY TOTAL			DAILY TOTAL	

DAILY CALORIES/ POINTS GOALS

WEEKLY EXERCISE TRACKER

SUNDAY	
FOODS	Calories/ Points
DAILY TOTAL	

ACTIVITY	
DISTANCE/DURATION/INTENSITY	CALORIES BURNED
TOTAL CALORIES BURNED	

MONDAY	−	=
TUESDAY	−	=
WEDNESDAY	−	=
THURSDAY	−	=
FRIDAY	−	=
SATURDAY	−	=
SUNDAY	−	=
WEEKLY CALORIES TOTALS	−	=
	Food	Exercise	Total

Weekly Meal Planner

DATE ___/___/___ TO ___/___/___

WEEKLY GOALS

1. _____ M T W T F S S
   □ □ □ □ □ □ □

2. _____ M T W T F S S
   □ □ □ □ □ □ □

3. _____ M T W T F S S
   □ □ □ □ □ □ □

MONDAY	
B	
L	
D	

TUESDAY	
B	
L	
D	

WEDNESDAY	
B	
L	
D	

THURSDAY	
B	
L	
D	

FRIDAY	
B	
L	
D	

SHOPPING LIST

- [ ] _____
- [ ] _____
- [ ] _____
- [ ] _____
- [ ] _____
- [ ] _____
- [ ] _____
- [ ] _____
- [ ] _____
- [ ] _____
- [ ] _____
- [ ] _____
- [ ] _____
- [ ] _____
- [ ] _____
- [ ] _____
- [ ] _____
- [ ] _____
- [ ] _____
- [ ] _____

> "Motivation is what gets you started. Habit is what keeps you going."
>
> JIM RYUN

NOTES

_____
_____
_____
_____
_____
_____
_____
_____
_____
_____

SATURDAY	
B	
L	
D	

SUNDAY	
B	
L	
D	

Calories/Points Tracker

DATE ____/____/____ TO ____/____/____

	MONDAY			TUESDAY	
	FOODS	Calories/ Points		FOODS	Calories/ Points
BREAKFAST					
LUNCH					
DINNER					
SNACKS					
	DAILY TOTAL			DAILY TOTAL	

WEDNESDAY		THURSDAY	
FOODS	Calories/ Points	FOODS	Calories/ Points
DAILY TOTAL		DAILY TOTAL	

Calories/Points Tracker

DATE ___ / ___ / ___ TO ___ / ___ / ___

	FRIDAY			SATURDAY	
	FOODS	Calories/Points		FOODS	Calories/Points
BREAKFAST					
LUNCH					
DINNER					
SNACKS					
	DAILY TOTAL			DAILY TOTAL	

WEEKLY EXERCISE TRACKER

ACTIVITY	
DISTANCE/DURATION/INTENSITY	CALORIES BURNED

SUNDAY	
FOODS	Calories/ Points
DAILY TOTAL	

TOTAL CALORIES BURNED	

MONDAY	-	=	
TUESDAY	-	=	
WEDNESDAY	-	=	
THURSDAY	-	=	
FRIDAY	-	=	
SATURDAY	-	=	
SUNDAY	-	=	
WEEKLY CALORIES TOTALS	-	=	
	Food	Exercise	Total

Weekly Meal Planner

DATE ___/___/___ TO ___/___/___

WEEKLY GOALS

1. _____ M T W T F S S
   ☐ ☐ ☐ ☐ ☐ ☐ ☐

2. _____ M T W T F S S
   ☐ ☐ ☐ ☐ ☐ ☐ ☐

3. _____ M T W T F S S
   ☐ ☐ ☐ ☐ ☐ ☐ ☐

MONDAY
B
L
D

TUESDAY
B
L
D

WEDNESDAY
B
L
D

THURSDAY
B
L
D

FRIDAY
B
L
D

- [ ] _____
- [ ] _____
- [ ] _____
- [ ] _____
- [ ] _____
- [ ] _____
- [ ] _____
- [ ] _____
- [ ] _____
- [ ] _____
- [ ] _____
- [ ] _____
- [ ] _____
- [ ] _____
- [ ] _____
- [ ] _____
- [ ] _____
- [ ] _____
- [ ] _____

> "Do one thing every day that scares you."
>
> MARY SCHMICH

NOTES

_____
_____
_____
_____
_____
_____
_____
_____
_____
_____
_____
_____
_____

SATURDAY	
B	
L	
D	

SUNDAY	
B	
L	
D	

Calories/Points Tracker

DATE ___ / ___ / ___ TO ___ / ___ / ___

	MONDAY			TUESDAY	
	FOODS	Calories/Points		FOODS	Calories/Points
BREAKFAST					
LUNCH					
DINNER					
SNACKS					
	DAILY TOTAL			DAILY TOTAL	

48

WEDNESDAY		THURSDAY	
FOODS	Calories/ Points	FOODS	Calories/ Points
DAILY TOTAL		DAILY TOTAL	

Breakfast BLT Salad

Salad for breakfast? Yes! This BLT-themed dish can be eaten anytime of the day, really, but eggs and bacon served over a simple massaged kale salad with avocado and tomatoes is a delicious, savory, healthy idea for starting your day.

SERVES 2

3 cups shredded stemmed lacinato kale

2 teaspoons extra-virgin olive oil

1 teaspoon red wine vinegar

¼ teaspoon plus a pinch of kosher salt

4 slices center-cut bacon, cooked and chopped

10 grape tomatoes, halved

2 ounces sliced avocado (½ small Hass)

2 large eggs, hard- or soft-boiled (see page 98), peeled and halved

Freshly ground black pepper

PER SERVING	1 salad
CALORIES	292
FAT	18 g
SATURATED FAT	4.5 g
CHOLESTEROL	191 mg
CARBOHYDRATE	18 g
FIBER	7 g
PROTEIN	18 g
SUGAR	3 g
SODIUM	336 mg

In a large bowl, combine the kale, olive oil, vinegar, and ¼ teaspoon of the salt. Massage with your hands until the kale softens, about 3 minutes.

Divide the kale between 2 bowls. Top each with the bacon, tomatoes, avocado, and eggs. Sprinkle with the remaining pinch of salt and pepper to taste, and serve.

Gluten-Free, Dairy-Free Blueberry Oatmeal Muffins

These muffins are insanely good—you'd never guess they are allergy-friendly.

MAKES 12 MUFFINS

Nonstick cooking spray

1½ cups gluten-free quick-cooking oats

1 cup unsweetened almond milk

⅔ cup gluten-free all-purpose flour mix

1 teaspoon baking powder

½ teaspoon baking soda

½ teaspoon kosher salt

½ cup packed light brown sugar

2 large egg whites

½ cup unsweetened applesauce

2 tablespoons honey

1 tablespoon coconut or canola oil

1 teaspoon vanilla extract

1 cup blueberries

PER SERVING	1 muffin
CALORIES	148
FAT	2.5 g
SATURATED FAT	0 g
CHOLESTEROL	0 mg
CARBOHYDRATE	33 g
FIBER	2.5 g
PROTEIN	3 g
SUGAR	18 g
SODIUM	169 mg

Preheat the oven to 400°F. Line 12 cups of a standard muffin tin with liners and spray lightly with nonstick spray.

Place the oats in a food processor and pulse a few times. Transfer the oats to a medium bowl, add the almond milk, and soak for about 30 minutes.

In a separate medium bowl, whisk together the flour mix, baking powder, baking soda, and salt.

In a large bowl, combine the brown sugar, egg whites, applesauce, honey, oil, and vanilla and mix well. Add the oat mixture and stir well. Slowly stir in the flour mixture and mix until just incorporated. Fold in the blueberries. Spoon the batter into the prepared muffin cups.

Bake until golden, 22 to 24 minutes.

Calories/Points Tracker

DATE ___/___/___ TO ___/___/___

	FRIDAY			SATURDAY	
	FOODS	Calories/ Points		FOODS	Calories/ Points
BREAKFAST					
LUNCH					
DINNER					
SNACKS					
	DAILY TOTAL			DAILY TOTAL	

DAILY CALORIES/ POINTS GOALS

WEEKLY EXERCISE TRACKER

SUNDAY	
FOODS	Calories/ Points
DAILY TOTAL	

ACTIVITY	
DISTANCE/DURATION/INTENSITY	CALORIES BURNED

TOTAL CALORIES BURNED	

MONDAY		-	=
TUESDAY		-	=
WEDNESDAY		-	=
THURSDAY		-	=
FRIDAY		-	=
SATURDAY		-	=
SUNDAY		-	=
WEEKLY CALORIES TOTALS		-	=
	Food	Exercise	Total

Weekly Meal Planner

DATE ____ / ____ / ____ TO ____ / ____ / ____

WEEKLY GOALS

1. _____ M T W T F S S
   ☐ ☐ ☐ ☐ ☐ ☐ ☐

2. _____ M T W T F S S
   ☐ ☐ ☐ ☐ ☐ ☐ ☐

3. _____ M T W T F S S
   ☐ ☐ ☐ ☐ ☐ ☐ ☐

MONDAY	
B	
L	
D	

TUESDAY	
B	
L	
D	

WEDNESDAY	
B	
L	
D	

THURSDAY	
B	
L	
D	

FRIDAY	
B	
L	
D	

SHOPPING LIST

- [ ] _____
- [ ] _____
- [ ] _____
- [ ] _____
- [ ] _____
- [ ] _____
- [ ] _____
- [ ] _____
- [ ] _____
- [ ] _____
- [ ] _____
- [ ] _____
- [ ] _____
- [ ] _____
- [ ] _____
- [ ] _____
- [ ] _____
- [ ] _____
- [ ] _____

superfood KIWIFRUIT

This small fuzzy fruit is pleasingly tart and has little seeds inside that are fun to crunch. Slice one into a fruit salad, or even scoop the flesh from the skin with a spoon for a snack!

NOTES

_____
_____
_____
_____
_____
_____
_____
_____
_____
_____

SATURDAY	
B	
L	
D	

SUNDAY	
B	
L	
D	

Calories/Points Tracker

	MONDAY			TUESDAY	
	FOODS	*Calories/ Points*		FOODS	*Calories/ Points*
BREAKFAST					
LUNCH					
DINNER					
SNACKS					
	DAILY TOTAL			DAILY TOTAL	

WEDNESDAY	
FOODS	Calories/ Points
DAILY TOTAL	

THURSDAY	
FOODS	Calories/ Points
DAILY TOTAL	

Calories/Points Tracker

DATE ___ / ___ / ___ TO ___ / ___ / ___

	FRIDAY			SATURDAY	
	FOODS	Calories/Points		FOODS	Calories/Points
BREAKFAST					
BREAKFAST					
BREAKFAST					
BREAKFAST					
BREAKFAST					
BREAKFAST					
LUNCH					
LUNCH					
LUNCH					
LUNCH					
LUNCH					
LUNCH					
LUNCH					
DINNER					
DINNER					
DINNER					
DINNER					
DINNER					
DINNER					
DINNER					
SNACKS					
SNACKS					
SNACKS					
	DAILY TOTAL			DAILY TOTAL	

WEEKLY EXERCISE TRACKER

SUNDAY	
FOODS	Calories/ Points
DAILY TOTAL	

ACTIVITY	
DISTANCE/DURATION/INTENSITY	CALORIES BURNED
TOTAL CALORIES BURNED	

MONDAY		–	=
TUESDAY		–	=
WEDNESDAY		–	=
THURSDAY		–	=
FRIDAY		–	=
SATURDAY		–	=
SUNDAY		–	=
WEEKLY CALORIES TOTALS	–	=	
	Food	Exercise	Total

Weekly Meal Planner

DATE ___/___/___ TO ___/___/___

WEEKLY GOALS

1. _____ M T W T F S S
   ☐ ☐ ☐ ☐ ☐ ☐ ☐

2. _____ M T W T F S S
   ☐ ☐ ☐ ☐ ☐ ☐ ☐

3. _____ M T W T F S S
   ☐ ☐ ☐ ☐ ☐ ☐ ☐

MONDAY	
B	
L	
D	

TUESDAY	
B	
L	
D	

WEDNESDAY	
B	
L	
D	

THURSDAY	
B	
L	
D	

FRIDAY	
B	
L	
D	

SHOPPING LIST

- [ ] _____
- [ ] _____
- [ ] _____
- [ ] _____
- [ ] _____
- [ ] _____
- [ ] _____
- [ ] _____
- [ ] _____
- [ ] _____
- [ ] _____
- [ ] _____
- [ ] _____
- [ ] _____
- [ ] _____
- [ ] _____
- [ ] _____
- [ ] _____
- [ ] _____
- [ ] _____

> "It does not matter how slowly you go as long as you do not stop."
>
> CONFUCIUS

NOTES

SATURDAY	
B	
L	
D	

SUNDAY	
B	
L	
D	

Calories/Points Tracker

DATE ___/___/___ TO ___/___/___

	MONDAY			TUESDAY	
	FOODS	Calories/Points		FOODS	Calories/Points
BREAKFAST					
LUNCH					
DINNER					
SNACKS					
	DAILY TOTAL			DAILY TOTAL	

WEDNESDAY			THURSDAY	
FOODS	Calories/ Points		FOODS	Calories/ Points
DAILY TOTAL			DAILY TOTAL	

Calories/Points Tracker

DATE ____/____/____ TO ____/____/____

	FRIDAY			SATURDAY	
	FOODS	Calories/Points		FOODS	Calories/Points
BREAKFAST					
LUNCH					
DINNER					
SNACKS					
	DAILY TOTAL			DAILY TOTAL	

WEEKLY EXERCISE TRACKER

ACTIVITY	
DISTANCE/DURATION/INTENSITY	CALORIES BURNED
TOTAL CALORIES BURNED	

SUNDAY	
FOODS	Calories/ Points
DAILY TOTAL	

		-	=	
MONDAY		-	=	
TUESDAY		-	=	
WEDNESDAY		-	=	
THURSDAY		-	=	
FRIDAY		-	=	
SATURDAY		-	=	
SUNDAY		-	=	
WEEKLY CALORIES TOTALS		-	=	
	Food	Exercise		Total

Weekly Meal Planner

DATE ____/____/____ TO ____/____/____

WEEKLY GOALS

1. _____ M T W T F S S
   ☐ ☐ ☐ ☐ ☐ ☐ ☐

2. _____ M T W T F S S
   ☐ ☐ ☐ ☐ ☐ ☐ ☐

3. _____ M T W T F S S
   ☐ ☐ ☐ ☐ ☐ ☐ ☐

MONDAY	
B	
L	
D	

TUESDAY	
B	
L	
D	

WEDNESDAY	
B	
L	
D	

THURSDAY	
B	
L	
D	

FRIDAY	
B	
L	
D	

SHOPPING LIST

- [ ] _____
- [ ] _____
- [ ] _____
- [ ] _____
- [ ] _____
- [ ] _____
- [ ] _____
- [ ] _____
- [ ] _____
- [ ] _____
- [ ] _____
- [ ] _____
- [ ] _____
- [ ] _____
- [ ] _____
- [ ] _____
- [ ] _____
- [ ] _____
- [ ] _____

superfood ORANGES

Widely available, this citrus is a great addition to a salad, and it's sweet enough to stand in for dessert.

NOTES

_____
_____
_____
_____
_____
_____
_____
_____
_____

SATURDAY	
B	
L	
D	

SUNDAY	
B	
L	
D	

Calories/Points Tracker

DATE _____ / _____ / _____ TO _____ / _____ / _____

	MONDAY			TUESDAY	
	FOODS	Calories/Points		FOODS	Calories/Points
BREAKFAST					
LUNCH					
DINNER					
SNACKS					
	DAILY TOTAL			DAILY TOTAL	

WEDNESDAY		THURSDAY	
FOODS	Calories/ Points	FOODS	Calories/ Points
DAILY TOTAL		DAILY TOTAL	

Calories/Points Tracker

DATE ___ / ___ / ___ TO ___ / ___ / ___

	FRIDAY			SATURDAY	
	FOODS	Calories/ Points		FOODS	Calories/ Points
BREAKFAST					
LUNCH					
DINNER					
SNACKS					
	DAILY TOTAL			DAILY TOTAL	

70

DAILY CALORIES/
POINTS GOALS

WEEKLY EXERCISE TRACKER

SUNDAY	
FOODS	Calories/ Points
DAILY TOTAL	

ACTIVITY	
DISTANCE/DURATION/INTENSITY	CALORIES BURNED
TOTAL CALORIES BURNED	

MONDAY	-	=
TUESDAY	-	=
WEDNESDAY	-	=
THURSDAY	-	=
FRIDAY	-	=
SATURDAY	-	=
SUNDAY	-	=
WEEKLY CALORIES TOTALS	-	=
	Food	Exercise	Total

Weekly Meal Planner

DATE ____ / ____ / ____ TO ____ / ____ / ____

WEEKLY GOALS

1. _____ M T W T F S S
   □ □ □ □ □ □ □

2. _____ M T W T F S S
   □ □ □ □ □ □ □

3. _____ M T W T F S S
   □ □ □ □ □ □ □

MONDAY
B
L
D

TUESDAY
B
L
D

WEDNESDAY
B
L
D

THURSDAY
B
L
D

FRIDAY
B
L
D

SHOPPING LIST

- [ ] _____
- [ ] _____
- [ ] _____
- [ ] _____
- [ ] _____
- [ ] _____
- [ ] _____
- [ ] _____
- [ ] _____
- [ ] _____
- [ ] _____
- [ ] _____
- [ ] _____
- [ ] _____
- [ ] _____
- [ ] _____
- [ ] _____
- [ ] _____
- [ ] _____

"Whether you believe
you can do a thing or
not, you are right."

HENRY FORD

NOTES

_____
_____
_____
_____
_____
_____
_____
_____
_____
_____
_____
_____

SATURDAY	
B	
L	
D	

SUNDAY	
B	
L	
D	

Skinny Overnight Oats in a Jar

A hearty, healthy breakfast packed with fiber, vitamins, and nutrients, these overnight oats require no cooking at all! I like to make a few jars to keep in the fridge for grabbing on my way out the door in the morning. I love to top this with pecans, but any other nut, as well as granola or cereal, is also great.

SERVES 1

¼ cup quick-cooking oats

½ cup unsweetened almond milk (or soy milk or fat-free dairy milk)

½ cup blueberries

¼ medium banana, sliced

½ tablespoon chia seeds

4 to 5 drops liquid stevia or sweetener of your choice (I like NuNaturals Vanilla)

Pinch of ground cinnamon

1 tablespoon chopped pecans (or any nut)

PER SERVING	1 jar
CALORIES	236
FAT	10 g
SATURATED FAT	.5 g
CHOLESTEROL	0 mg
CARBOHYDRATE	35 g
FIBER	8.5 g
PROTEIN	6 g
SUGAR	12 g
SODIUM	95 mg

In a jar, combine the oats, milk, blueberries, banana, chia seeds, sweetener, and cinnamon. Shake well, cover, and refrigerate overnight.

The next morning, top with the pecans and enjoy.

PB&J Smoothie

My favorite smoothie order at my gym includes strawberries, blueberries, peanut butter, and almond milk. It tastes almost like peanut butter and grape jelly, even though it doesn't have any grapes. I often make this myself at home; the peanut butter is a great source of protein and keeps me full until lunch. And I just love how it tastes!

SERVES 1

¾ cup fresh or frozen blueberries

¾ cup sliced fresh strawberries

¾ cup unsweetened vanilla almond milk

1 tablespoon smooth peanut butter

5 to 6 drops liquid stevia or sweetener of your choice

¼ cup ice

In a blender, combine the blueberries, strawberries, almond milk, peanut butter, sweetener, and ice. Blend until smooth and enjoy immediately.

PER SERVING	1 smoothie
CALORIES	222
FAT	11 g
SATURATED FAT	1.5 g
CHOLESTEROL	0 mg
CARBOHYDRATE	29 g
FIBER	7.5 g
PROTEIN	6 g
SUGAR	19 g
SODIUM	216 mg

Calories/Points Tracker

DATE ___ / ___ / ___ TO ___ / ___ / ___

	MONDAY			TUESDAY	
	FOODS	Calories/Points		FOODS	Calories/Points
BREAKFAST					
LUNCH					
DINNER					
SNACKS					
	DAILY TOTAL			DAILY TOTAL	

WEDNESDAY			THURSDAY	
FOODS	Calories/ Points		FOODS	Calories/ Points
DAILY TOTAL			DAILY TOTAL	

Calories/Points Tracker

DATE ___/___/___ TO ___/___/___

	FRIDAY			SATURDAY	
	FOODS	Calories/ Points		FOODS	Calories/ Points
BREAKFAST					
LUNCH					
DINNER					
SNACKS					
	DAILY TOTAL			DAILY TOTAL	

WEEKLY EXERCISE TRACKER

ACTIVITY		
DISTANCE/DURATION/INTENSITY		CALORIES BURNED

SUNDAY	
FOODS	Calories/ Points
DAILY TOTAL	

TOTAL CALORIES BURNED	

MONDAY	-	=	
TUESDAY	-	=	
WEDNESDAY	-	=	
THURSDAY	-	=	
FRIDAY	-	=	
SATURDAY	-	=	
SUNDAY	-	=	
WEEKLY CALORIES TOTALS	-	=	
	Food	Exercise	Total

Weekly Meal Planner

DATE ___ / ___ / ___ TO ___ / ___ / ___

WEEKLY GOALS

1. _____ M T W T F S S
   ☐ ☐ ☐ ☐ ☐ ☐ ☐

2. _____ M T W T F S S
   ☐ ☐ ☐ ☐ ☐ ☐ ☐

3. _____ M T W T F S S
   ☐ ☐ ☐ ☐ ☐ ☐ ☐

MONDAY
B
L
D

TUESDAY
B
L
D

WEDNESDAY
B
L
D

THURSDAY
B
L
D

FRIDAY
B
L
D

SHOPPING LIST

- [ ] _____
- [ ] _____
- [ ] _____
- [ ] _____
- [ ] _____
- [ ] _____
- [ ] _____
- [ ] _____
- [ ] _____
- [ ] _____
- [ ] _____
- [ ] _____
- [ ] _____
- [ ] _____
- [ ] _____
- [ ] _____
- [ ] _____
- [ ] _____
- [ ] _____
- [ ] _____

> "Success is not the key to happiness. Happiness is the key to success."
>
> ALBERT SCHWEITZER

NOTES

_____
_____
_____
_____
_____
_____
_____
_____
_____
_____
_____
_____

SATURDAY	
B	
L	
D	

SUNDAY	
B	
L	
D	

Calories/Points Tracker

DATE ___/___/___ TO ___/___/___

	MONDAY			TUESDAY	
	FOODS	Calories/Points		FOODS	Calories/Points
BREAKFAST					
LUNCH					
DINNER					
SNACKS					
	DAILY TOTAL			DAILY TOTAL	

WEDNESDAY		THURSDAY	
FOODS	Calories/ Points	FOODS	Calories/ Points
DAILY TOTAL		DAILY TOTAL	

Calories/Points Tracker

DATE ___/___/___ TO ___/___/___

	FRIDAY			SATURDAY	
	FOODS	Calories/Points		FOODS	Calories/Points
BREAKFAST					
LUNCH					
DINNER					
SNACKS					
	DAILY TOTAL			DAILY TOTAL	

DAILY CALORIES/ POINTS GOALS

WEEKLY EXERCISE TRACKER

SUNDAY	
FOODS	Calories/ Points
DAILY TOTAL	

ACTIVITY	
DISTANCE/DURATION/INTENSITY	CALORIES BURNED
TOTAL CALORIES BURNED	

	Food	Exercise	Total
MONDAY		−	=
TUESDAY		−	=
WEDNESDAY		−	=
THURSDAY		−	=
FRIDAY		−	=
SATURDAY		−	=
SUNDAY		−	=
WEEKLY CALORIES TOTALS		−	=

Weekly Meal Planner

DATE ____ / ____ / ____ TO ____ / ____ / ____

WEEKLY GOALS

1. _____ M T W T F S S ☐☐☐☐☐☐☐

2. _____ M T W T F S S ☐☐☐☐☐☐☐

3. _____ M T W T F S S ☐☐☐☐☐☐☐

MONDAY	
B	
L	
D	

TUESDAY	
B	
L	
D	

WEDNESDAY	
B	
L	
D	

THURSDAY	
B	
L	
D	

FRIDAY	
B	
L	
D	

- [ ] _____
- [ ] _____
- [ ] _____
- [ ] _____
- [ ] _____
- [ ] _____
- [ ] _____
- [ ] _____
- [ ] _____
- [ ] _____
- [ ] _____
- [ ] _____
- [ ] _____
- [ ] _____
- [ ] _____
- [ ] _____
- [ ] _____
- [ ] _____
- [ ] _____

superfood MUSHROOMS

You will reap nutritional benefits from any type of mushroom. Sauté some until golden brown, and add to pastas, egg dishes, or serve as a side dish.

NOTES

_____
_____
_____
_____
_____
_____
_____
_____
_____

SATURDAY	
B	
L	
D	

SUNDAY	
B	
L	
D	

Calories/Points Tracker

DATE ___/___/___ TO ___/___/___

	MONDAY			TUESDAY	
	FOODS	Calories/Points		FOODS	Calories/Points
BREAKFAST					
LUNCH					
DINNER					
SNACKS					
	DAILY TOTAL			DAILY TOTAL	

WEDNESDAY	
FOODS	Calories/ Points
DAILY TOTAL	

THURSDAY	
FOODS	Calories/ Points
DAILY TOTAL	

Calories/Points Tracker

DATE ___ / ___ / ___ TO ___ / ___ / ___

	FRIDAY			SATURDAY	
	FOODS	Calories/Points		FOODS	Calories/Points
BREAKFAST					
LUNCH					
DINNER					
SNACKS					
	DAILY TOTAL			DAILY TOTAL	

WEEKLY EXERCISE TRACKER

SUNDAY	
FOODS	Calories/ Points
DAILY TOTAL	

ACTIVITY	
DISTANCE/DURATION/INTENSITY	CALORIES BURNED
TOTAL CALORIES BURNED	

MONDAY	-	=	
TUESDAY	-	=	
WEDNESDAY	-	=	
THURSDAY	-	=	
FRIDAY	-	=	
SATURDAY	-	=	
SUNDAY	-	=	
WEEKLY CALORIES TOTALS	-	=	
	Food	Exercise	Total

Weekly Meal Planner

DATE ___ / ___ / ___ TO ___ / ___ / ___

WEEKLY GOALS

1. _____ M T W T F S S
                                                     ☐ ☐ ☐ ☐ ☐ ☐ ☐

2. _____ M T W T F S S
                                                     ☐ ☐ ☐ ☐ ☐ ☐ ☐

3. _____ M T W T F S S
                                                     ☐ ☐ ☐ ☐ ☐ ☐ ☐

MONDAY
B
L
D

TUESDAY
B
L
D

WEDNESDAY
B
L
D

THURSDAY
B
L
D

FRIDAY
B
L
D

SHOPPING LIST

- [ ] _____
- [ ] _____
- [ ] _____
- [ ] _____
- [ ] _____
- [ ] _____
- [ ] _____
- [ ] _____
- [ ] _____
- [ ] _____
- [ ] _____
- [ ] _____
- [ ] _____
- [ ] _____
- [ ] _____
- [ ] _____
- [ ] _____
- [ ] _____
- [ ] _____
- [ ] _____

> "Nothing is impossible,
> the word itself says,
> 'I'm possible'!"
>
> AUDREY HEPBURN

NOTES

_____
_____
_____
_____
_____
_____
_____
_____
_____
_____
_____
_____
_____
_____

SATURDAY	
B	
L	
D	

SUNDAY	
B	
L	
D	

Calories/Points Tracker

DATE _____ / _____ / _____ TO _____ / _____ / _____

	MONDAY			TUESDAY	
	FOODS	Calories/Points		FOODS	Calories/Points
BREAKFAST					
LUNCH					
DINNER					
SNACKS					
	DAILY TOTAL			DAILY TOTAL	

WEDNESDAY			THURSDAY	
FOODS	Calories/Points		FOODS	Calories/Points
DAILY TOTAL			DAILY TOTAL	

Calories/Points Tracker

DATE ___ / ___ / ___ TO ___ / ___ / ___

	FRIDAY			SATURDAY	
	FOODS	Calories/ Points		FOODS	Calories/ Points
BREAKFAST					
LUNCH					
DINNER					
SNACKS					
	DAILY TOTAL			DAILY TOTAL	

WEEKLY EXERCISE TRACKER

SUNDAY	
FOODS	Calories/ Points
DAILY TOTAL	

ACTIVITY	
DISTANCE/DURATION/INTENSITY	CALORIES BURNED
TOTAL CALORIES BURNED	

MONDAY		-	=
TUESDAY		-	=
WEDNESDAY		-	=
THURSDAY		-	=
FRIDAY		-	=
SATURDAY		-	=
SUNDAY		-	=
WEEKLY CALORIES TOTALS	Food	Exercise	Total

How to Make Perfect Hard-Boiled Eggs in the Instant Pot®

The Instant Pot® (a brand of electric pressure cooker) is my favorite tool for cooking eggs because it's so fast and the eggs peel very easily after they are cooked. I love to keep several hard-boiled eggs in my refrigerator to use for breakfasts on the go, to toss in salads, for topping avocado toast, and so many other quick meals. My simple formula will give you perfect, easy-to-peel eggs every time. The cooked eggs will keep in the refrigerator for 4 to 5 days, and you can easily double the number of eggs, leaving the water and cook time the same.

MAKES 4 EGGS · SERVES 4

1 cup water

4 large eggs

Place the steamer rack that came with the pressure cooker in the bottom of the pot. Pour in the water. Place the eggs on the rack.

Cook on high pressure on manual for 5 minutes. Use natural release for 5 minutes, then quick release (place a towel over the valve to contain the steam). Carefully remove the eggs from the pressure cooker. Quickly run the eggs under cold water until they are cool enough to handle. Peel right away.

NOTE: *For soft-boiled eggs, proceed as directed, but cook on high pressure on manual for 3 minutes and use quick release.*

PER SERVING	1 egg
CALORIES	72
FAT	5 g
SATURATED FAT	1.5 g
CHOLESTEROL	186 mg
CARBOHYDRATE	0 g
FIBER	0 g
PROTEIN	6 g
SUGAR	0 g
SODIUM	71 mg

Loaded Baked Omelet Muffins

These mini, savory muffins were inspired by meals I enjoyed during a vacation to Beaches Resort in Ocho Rios, Jamaica, where every morning I would get an omelet chock-full of vegetables. I created this easy, make-ahead recipe so I can have a delicious, healthy breakfast no matter how hectic the day may be. I used some of my favorite omelet ingredients, but you can switch it up and add whatever you like or have on hand.

MAKES 12 OMELET MUFFINS · SERVES 6

Nonstick cooking spray

6 large eggs

6 large egg whites

¼ teaspoon kosher salt

Freshly ground black pepper

3 slices bacon, cooked and chopped

3 tablespoons thawed frozen spinach, drained

3 tablespoons finely chopped tomato

3 tablespoons finely chopped onion

3 tablespoons finely chopped bell pepper

2 ounces shredded cheddar cheese

PER SERVING	2 omelet muffins
CALORIES	147
FAT	9 g
SATURATED FAT	3.5 g
CHOLESTEROL	196 mg
CARBOHYDRATE	3 g
FIBER	.5 g
PROTEIN	14 g
SUGAR	0 g
SODIUM	287 mg

Preheat the oven to 350°F. Coat 12 cups of a standard muffin tin with cooking spray.

In a large bowl, whisk together the whole eggs, egg whites, salt, and black pepper to taste. Stir in the bacon, spinach, tomato, onion, bell pepper, and cheddar. Divide the mixture among the prepared muffin cups.

Place the muffin tin on a baking sheet and bake until set, 20 to 25 minutes.

Weekly Meal Planner

DATE _____ / _____ / _____ TO _____ / _____ / _____

WEEKLY GOALS

1. _____ M T W T F S S
   ☐ ☐ ☐ ☐ ☐ ☐ ☐

2. _____ M T W T F S S
   ☐ ☐ ☐ ☐ ☐ ☐ ☐

3. _____ M T W T F S S
   ☐ ☐ ☐ ☐ ☐ ☐ ☐

MONDAY	
B	
L	
D	

TUESDAY	
B	
L	
D	

WEDNESDAY	
B	
L	
D	

THURSDAY	
B	
L	
D	

FRIDAY	
B	
L	
D	

- ☐ _____
- ☐ _____
- ☐ _____
- ☐ _____
- ☐ _____
- ☐ _____
- ☐ _____
- ☐ _____
- ☐ _____
- ☐ _____
- ☐ _____
- ☐ _____
- ☐ _____
- ☐ _____
- ☐ _____
- ☐ _____
- ☐ _____
- ☐ _____
- ☐ _____
- ☐ _____

superfood CHERRIES

Summer is the season for cherries. Snack on them plain, toss them into salads, or make a sauce with them for pork, which is delicious paired with fruit.

NOTES

_____

_____

_____

_____

_____

_____

_____

_____

_____

_____

_____

_____

SATURDAY	
B	
L	
D	

SUNDAY	
B	
L	
D	

Calories/Points Tracker

DATE ___ / ___ / ___ TO ___ / ___ / ___

	MONDAY			TUESDAY	
	FOODS	Calories/ Points		FOODS	Calories/ Points
BREAKFAST					
LUNCH					
DINNER					
SNACKS					
	DAILY TOTAL			DAILY TOTAL	

WEDNESDAY		THURSDAY	
FOODS	Calories/ Points	FOODS	Calories/ Points
DAILY TOTAL		DAILY TOTAL	

Calories/Points Tracker

	FRIDAY			SATURDAY	
	FOODS	Calories/ Points		FOODS	Calories/ Points
BREAKFAST					
LUNCH					
DINNER					
SNACKS					
	DAILY TOTAL			DAILY TOTAL	

WEEKLY EXERCISE TRACKER

ACTIVITY	
DISTANCE/DURATION/INTENSITY	CALORIES BURNED

SUNDAY

FOODS	Calories/ Points
DAILY TOTAL	

TOTAL CALORIES BURNED	

MONDAY		-	=
TUESDAY		-	=
WEDNESDAY		-	=
THURSDAY		-	=
FRIDAY		-	=
SATURDAY		-	=
SUNDAY		-	=
WEEKLY CALORIES TOTALS	-	=	
	Food	Exercise	Total

Weekly Meal Planner

DATE ____/____/____ TO ____/____/____

WEEKLY GOALS

1. _____ M T W T F S S
   ☐ ☐ ☐ ☐ ☐ ☐ ☐

2. _____ M T W T F S S
   ☐ ☐ ☐ ☐ ☐ ☐ ☐

3. _____ M T W T F S S
   ☐ ☐ ☐ ☐ ☐ ☐ ☐

MONDAY	
B	
L	
D	

TUESDAY	
B	
L	
D	

WEDNESDAY	
B	
L	
D	

THURSDAY	
B	
L	
D	

FRIDAY	
B	
L	
D	

SHOPPING LIST

☐ _____
☐ _____
☐ _____
☐ _____
☐ _____
☐ _____
☐ _____
☐ _____
☐ _____
☐ _____
☐ _____
☐ _____
☐ _____
☐ _____
☐ _____
☐ _____
☐ _____
☐ _____
☐ _____

> "We are what we
> repeatedly do."
>
> ARISTOTLE

NOTES

_____
_____
_____
_____
_____
_____
_____
_____
_____
_____
_____
_____

SATURDAY	
B	
L	
D	

SUNDAY	
B	
L	
D	

Calories/Points Tracker

DATE _____ / _____ / _____ TO _____ / _____ / _____

	MONDAY			TUESDAY	
	FOODS	Calories/Points		FOODS	Calories/Points
BREAKFAST					
LUNCH					
DINNER					
SNACKS					
	DAILY TOTAL			DAILY TOTAL	

WEDNESDAY		THURSDAY	
FOODS	Calories/Points	FOODS	Calories/Points
DAILY TOTAL		DAILY TOTAL	

Calories/Points Tracker

DATE ___/___/___ TO ___/___/___

	FRIDAY			SATURDAY	
	FOODS	Calories/ Points		FOODS	Calories/ Points
BREAKFAST					
LUNCH					
DINNER					
SNACKS					
	DAILY TOTAL			DAILY TOTAL	

DAILY CALORIES/ POINTS GOALS

WEEKLY EXERCISE TRACKER

SUNDAY	
FOODS	Calories/ Points
DAILY TOTAL	

ACTIVITY		
DISTANCE/DURATION/INTENSITY		CALORIES BURNED
TOTAL CALORIES BURNED		

MONDAY		–	=
TUESDAY		–	=
WEDNESDAY		–	=
THURSDAY		–	=
FRIDAY		–	=
SATURDAY		–	=
SUNDAY		–	=
WEEKLY CALORIES TOTALS		–	=
	Food	Exercise	Total

111

Weekly Meal Planner

DATE ____ / ____ / ____ TO ____ / ____ / ____

1. _____ M T W T F S S
   ☐☐☐☐☐☐☐

2. _____ M T W T F S S
   ☐☐☐☐☐☐☐

3. _____ M T W T F S S
   ☐☐☐☐☐☐☐

MONDAY	
B	
L	
D	

TUESDAY	
B	
L	
D	

WEDNESDAY	
B	
L	
D	

THURSDAY	
B	
L	
D	

FRIDAY	
B	
L	
D	

SHOPPING LIST

- [ ] _____
- [ ] _____
- [ ] _____
- [ ] _____
- [ ] _____
- [ ] _____
- [ ] _____
- [ ] _____
- [ ] _____
- [ ] _____
- [ ] _____
- [ ] _____
- [ ] _____
- [ ] _____
- [ ] _____
- [ ] _____
- [ ] _____
- [ ] _____
- [ ] _____

> "Keep your face always toward the sunshine— and shadows will fall behind you."
>
> **WALT WHITMAN**

NOTES

_____
_____
_____
_____
_____
_____
_____
_____
_____
_____
_____
_____
_____

SATURDAY	
B	
L	
D	

SUNDAY	
B	
L	
D	

Calories/Points Tracker

DATE ___ / ___ / ___ TO ___ / ___ / ___

	MONDAY			TUESDAY	
	FOODS	Calories/ Points		FOODS	Calories/ Points
BREAKFAST					
LUNCH					
DINNER					
SNACKS					
	DAILY TOTAL			DAILY TOTAL	

WEDNESDAY		THURSDAY	
FOODS	Calories/Points	FOODS	Calories/Points
DAILY TOTAL		DAILY TOTAL	

Calories/Points Tracker

DATE ___ / ___ / ___ TO ___ / ___ / ___

	FRIDAY			SATURDAY	
	FOODS	Calories/ Points		FOODS	Calories/ Points
BREAKFAST					
LUNCH					
DINNER					
SNACKS					
	DAILY TOTAL			DAILY TOTAL	

WEEKLY EXERCISE TRACKER

SUNDAY	
FOODS	Calories/ Points
DAILY TOTAL	

ACTIVITY		
DISTANCE/DURATION/INTENSITY		CALORIES BURNED
TOTAL CALORIES BURNED		

MONDAY	-	=
TUESDAY	-	=
WEDNESDAY	-	=
THURSDAY	-	=
FRIDAY	-	=
SATURDAY	-	=
SUNDAY	-	=
WEEKLY CALORIES TOTALS	-	=
	Food	Exercise	Total

Weekly Meal Planner

DATE _____ / _____ / _____ TO _____ / _____ / _____

WEEKLY GOALS

1. _____
M T W T F S S
☐ ☐ ☐ ☐ ☐ ☐ ☐

2. _____
M T W T F S S
☐ ☐ ☐ ☐ ☐ ☐ ☐

3. _____
M T W T F S S
☐ ☐ ☐ ☐ ☐ ☐ ☐

MONDAY	
B	
L	
D	

TUESDAY	
B	
L	
D	

WEDNESDAY	
B	
L	
D	

THURSDAY	
B	
L	
D	

FRIDAY	
B	
L	
D	

☐ _____

☐ _____

☐ _____

☐ _____

☐ _____

☐ _____

☐ _____

☐ _____

☐ _____

☐ _____

☐ _____

☐ _____

☐ _____

☐ _____

☐ _____

☐ _____

☐ _____

☐ _____

superfood
SWEET POTATOES

Trust me when I say that roasting sweet potatoes is the way to go! Microwaving will get them cooked, but the caramelization that comes through roasting is worth the extra time.

NOTES

_____

_____

_____

_____

_____

_____

_____

_____

_____

SATURDAY	
B	
L	
D	

SUNDAY	
B	
L	
D	

Calories/Points Tracker

DATE _____ / _____ / _____ TO _____ / _____ / _____

	MONDAY			TUESDAY	
	FOODS	Calories/Points		FOODS	Calories/Points
BREAKFAST					
LUNCH					
DINNER					
SNACKS					
	DAILY TOTAL			DAILY TOTAL	

WEDNESDAY			THURSDAY	
FOODS	Calories/ Points		FOODS	Calories/ Points
DAILY TOTAL			DAILY TOTAL	

Hummus Avocado Toast

This simple, vegan toast is perfect for breakfast or lunch! Ready in less than 5 minutes, with good-for-you whole grains, protein, vitamins, and antioxidants—what could be better?

SERVES 1

- 2 tablespoons hummus
- 2 (1-ounce) slices whole-grain bread, toasted
- 6 thin cucumber slices
- 1 small radish, thinly sliced
- 1 ounce avocado, thinly sliced (¼ small Hass)
- ⅛ teaspoon kosher salt
- Crushed red pepper flakes
- Freshly ground black pepper
- ¼ cup baby arugula
- 1 lemon wedge

PER SERVING	2 toasts
CALORIES	255
FAT	9.5 g
SATURATED FAT	1.5 g
CHOLESTEROL	0 mg
CARBOHYDRATE	35 g
FIBER	9.5 g
PROTEIN	11 g
SUGAR	4.5 g
SODIUM	474 mg

Spread the hummus onto the toast. Top with the cucumber, radish, and avocado slices. Sprinkle with the salt. Season with pepper flakes and black pepper to taste. Top with the arugula and squeeze the lemon wedge over the arugula. Serve.

French Bread Pizza Caprese

When my garden is overflowing with tomatoes and basil during the summer, I take advantage by making these simple French bread pizzas. Only 5 ingredients, less than 10 minutes to make, and so delicious! You can also make these on a grill or in a toaster.

SERVES 4

1 (8-ounce) whole wheat French baguette

4 ounces fresh mozzarella cheese, thinly sliced

2 medium tomatoes, thinly sliced

1 tablespoon balsamic glaze

1 tablespoon chopped fresh basil

PER SERVING	1 pizza
CALORIES	252
FAT	9 g
SATURATED FAT	4 g
CHOLESTEROL	22 mg
CARBOHYDRATE	33 g
FIBER	4 g
PROTEIN	12 g
SUGAR	6 g
SODIUM	483 mg

Preheat a broiler.

Halve the bread lengthwise horizontally, then cut each half crosswise into 2 pieces to give you 4 pieces total. Arrange the bread cut side up on a baking sheet. Tear the cheese into pieces and arrange it on top of the bread.

Broil until the cheese melts, 2 to 3 minutes.

Remove the baking sheet from the oven. Top the pizzas with the tomatoes, drizzle with the balsamic glaze, and sprinkle with the basil. Serve.

Calories/Points Tracker

DATE ___/___/___ TO ___/___/___

	FRIDAY			SATURDAY	
	FOODS	Calories/ Points		FOODS	Calories/ Points
BREAKFAST					
LUNCH					
DINNER					
SNACKS					
	DAILY TOTAL			DAILY TOTAL	

WEEKLY EXERCISE TRACKER

ACTIVITY	
DISTANCE/DURATION/INTENSITY	CALORIES BURNED

SUNDAY	
FOODS	Calories/ Points
DAILY TOTAL	

TOTAL CALORIES BURNED		

MONDAY	−	=	
TUESDAY	−	=	
WEDNESDAY	−	=	
THURSDAY	−	=	
FRIDAY	−	=	
SATURDAY	−	=	
SUNDAY	−	=	
WEEKLY CALORIES TOTALS	−	=	
	Food	Exercise	Total

Weekly Meal Planner

DATE ___/___/___ TO ___/___/___

WEEKLY GOALS

1. _____   M T W T F S S
   ☐ ☐ ☐ ☐ ☐ ☐ ☐

2. _____   M T W T F S S
   ☐ ☐ ☐ ☐ ☐ ☐ ☐

3. _____   M T W T F S S
   ☐ ☐ ☐ ☐ ☐ ☐ ☐

MONDAY	
B	
L	
D	

TUESDAY	
B	
L	
D	

WEDNESDAY	
B	
L	
D	

THURSDAY	
B	
L	
D	

FRIDAY	
B	
L	
D	

SHOPPING LIST

- [ ] _____
- [ ] _____
- [ ] _____
- [ ] _____
- [ ] _____
- [ ] _____
- [ ] _____
- [ ] _____
- [ ] _____
- [ ] _____
- [ ] _____
- [ ] _____
- [ ] _____
- [ ] _____
- [ ] _____
- [ ] _____
- [ ] _____
- [ ] _____
- [ ] _____

> "Whatever the mind of man can conceive and believe, it can achieve."
>
> NAPOLEON HILL

NOTES

_____
_____
_____
_____
_____
_____
_____
_____
_____
_____
_____

SATURDAY	
B	
L	
D	

SUNDAY	
B	
L	
D	

Calories/Points Tracker

	MONDAY			TUESDAY	
	FOODS	Calories/ Points		FOODS	Calories/ Points
BREAKFAST					
LUNCH					
DINNER					
SNACKS					
	DAILY TOTAL			DAILY TOTAL	

WEDNESDAY		THURSDAY	
FOODS	Calories/ Points	FOODS	Calories/ Points
DAILY TOTAL		DAILY TOTAL	

Calories/Points Tracker

DATE ___ / ___ / ___ TO ___ / ___ / ___

	FRIDAY			SATURDAY	
	FOODS	Calories/ Points		FOODS	Calories/ Points
BREAKFAST					
LUNCH					
DINNER					
SNACKS					
	DAILY TOTAL			DAILY TOTAL	

WEEKLY EXERCISE TRACKER

SUNDAY	
FOODS	Calories/ Points
DAILY TOTAL	

ACTIVITY	
DISTANCE/DURATION/INTENSITY	CALORIES BURNED
TOTAL CALORIES BURNED	

MONDAY		–		=
TUESDAY		–		=
WEDNESDAY		–		=
THURSDAY		–		=
FRIDAY		–		=
SATURDAY		–		=
SUNDAY		–		=
WEEKLY CALORIES TOTALS		–		=
	Food	Exercise		Total

Weekly Meal Planner

DATE ___/___/___ TO ___/___/___

WEEKLY GOALS

1. _____ M T W T F S S
   ☐ ☐ ☐ ☐ ☐ ☐ ☐

2. _____ M T W T F S S
   ☐ ☐ ☐ ☐ ☐ ☐ ☐

3. _____ M T W T F S S
   ☐ ☐ ☐ ☐ ☐ ☐ ☐

MONDAY	
B	
L	
D	

TUESDAY	
B	
L	
D	

WEDNESDAY	
B	
L	
D	

THURSDAY	
B	
L	
D	

FRIDAY	
B	
L	
D	

☐ _____

☐ _____

☐ _____

☐ _____

☐ _____

☐ _____

☐ _____

☐ _____

☐ _____

☐ _____

☐ _____

☐ _____

☐ _____

☐ _____

☐ _____

☐ _____

☐ _____

☐ _____

☐ _____

superfood EGGS

The most versatile food, eggs have a zillion preparations. Hard-boiled, poached, scrambled—there's no excuse for not eating this healthy food!

NOTES

_____

_____

_____

_____

_____

_____

_____

_____

_____

_____

_____

_____

SATURDAY	
B	
L	
D	

SUNDAY	
B	
L	
D	

Calories/Points Tracker

DATE _____ / _____ / _____ TO _____ / _____ / _____

	MONDAY			TUESDAY	
	FOODS	Calories/Points		FOODS	Calories/Points
BREAKFAST					
LUNCH					
DINNER					
SNACKS					
	DAILY TOTAL			DAILY TOTAL	

WEDNESDAY		THURSDAY	
FOODS	Calories/ Points	FOODS	Calories/ Points
DAILY TOTAL		DAILY TOTAL	

Calories/Points Tracker

DATE ___ / ___ / ___ TO ___ / ___ / ___

	FRIDAY			SATURDAY	
	FOODS	Calories/Points		FOODS	Calories/Points
BREAKFAST					
LUNCH					
DINNER					
SNACKS					
	DAILY TOTAL			DAILY TOTAL	

DAILY CALORIES/
POINTS GOALS

WEEKLY EXERCISE TRACKER

SUNDAY	
FOODS	Calories/ Points
DAILY TOTAL	

ACTIVITY	
DISTANCE/DURATION/INTENSITY	CALORIES BURNED
TOTAL CALORIES BURNED	

MONDAY	-	=
TUESDAY	-	=
WEDNESDAY	-	=
THURSDAY	-	=
FRIDAY	-	=
SATURDAY	-	=
SUNDAY	-	=
WEEKLY CALORIES TOTALS	-	=
	Food	Exercise	Total

Weekly Meal Planner

DATE _____ / _____ / _____ TO _____ / _____ / _____

1. _____ M T W T F S S ☐☐☐☐☐☐☐

2. _____ M T W T F S S ☐☐☐☐☐☐☐

3. _____ M T W T F S S ☐☐☐☐☐☐☐

MONDAY	
B	
L	
D	

TUESDAY	
B	
L	
D	

WEDNESDAY	
B	
L	
D	

THURSDAY	
B	
L	
D	

FRIDAY	
B	
L	
D	

SHOPPING LIST

- [ ] _____
- [ ] _____
- [ ] _____
- [ ] _____
- [ ] _____
- [ ] _____
- [ ] _____
- [ ] _____
- [ ] _____
- [ ] _____
- [ ] _____
- [ ] _____
- [ ] _____
- [ ] _____
- [ ] _____
- [ ] _____
- [ ] _____
- [ ] _____
- [ ] _____

> "The most difficult thing is the decision to act, the rest is merely tenacity."
>
> AMELIA EARHART

NOTES

_____
_____
_____
_____
_____
_____
_____
_____
_____
_____

SATURDAY	
B	
L	
D	

SUNDAY	
B	
L	
D	

Calories/Points Tracker

DATE ____ / ___ / ___ TO ____ / ___ / ___

	MONDAY			TUESDAY	
	FOODS	Calories/ Points		FOODS	Calories/ Points
BREAKFAST					
LUNCH					
DINNER					
SNACKS					
	DAILY TOTAL			DAILY TOTAL	

WEDNESDAY		THURSDAY	
FOODS	Calories/ Points	FOODS	Calories/ Points
DAILY TOTAL		DAILY TOTAL	

Calories/Points Tracker

DATE ___/___/___ TO ___/___/___

	FRIDAY			SATURDAY	
	FOODS	Calories/Points		FOODS	Calories/Points
BREAKFAST					
LUNCH					
DINNER					
SNACKS					
	DAILY TOTAL			DAILY TOTAL	

WEEKLY EXERCISE TRACKER

SUNDAY	
FOODS	Calories/ Points
DAILY TOTAL	

ACTIVITY	
DISTANCE/DURATION/INTENSITY	CALORIES BURNED
TOTAL CALORIES BURNED	

MONDAY		-	=
TUESDAY		-	=
WEDNESDAY		-	=
THURSDAY		-	=
FRIDAY		-	=
SATURDAY		-	=
SUNDAY		-	=
WEEKLY CALORIES TOTALS	-	=	
	Food	Exercise	Total

Weekly Meal Planner

DATE ___ / ___ / ___ TO ___ / ___ / ___

WEEKLY GOALS

1. _____ M T W T F S S
   ☐ ☐ ☐ ☐ ☐ ☐ ☐

2. _____ M T W T F S S
   ☐ ☐ ☐ ☐ ☐ ☐ ☐

3. _____ M T W T F S S
   ☐ ☐ ☐ ☐ ☐ ☐ ☐

MONDAY	
B	
L	
D	

TUESDAY	
B	
L	
D	

WEDNESDAY	
B	
L	
D	

THURSDAY	
B	
L	
D	

FRIDAY	
B	
L	
D	

SHOPPING LIST

- [ ] _____
- [ ] _____
- [ ] _____
- [ ] _____
- [ ] _____
- [ ] _____
- [ ] _____
- [ ] _____
- [ ] _____
- [ ] _____
- [ ] _____
- [ ] _____
- [ ] _____
- [ ] _____
- [ ] _____
- [ ] _____
- [ ] _____
- [ ] _____
- [ ] _____

> "I am not a product of my circumstances. I am a product of my decisions."
>
> STEPHEN R. COVEY

NOTES

SATURDAY	
B	
L	
D	

SUNDAY	
B	
L	
D	

Sheet-Pan Italian Chicken and Veggie Dinner

This meal, made with colorful vegetables and boneless, skinless chicken thighs (which are much juicier than breasts) all tossed with a simple Italian dressing marinade, can be marinated ahead of time and roasted just before dinner. If you want to include grains, quinoa or brown rice would be a great addition.

SERVES 4

MARINADE

- 3 tablespoons olive oil
- 2 tablespoons red wine vinegar
- 1 garlic clove, crushed with the side of a knife
- 1 teaspoon kosher salt
- ½ teaspoon onion powder
- ½ teaspoon dried oregano
- ½ teaspoon dried basil
- ¼ teaspoon dried thyme
- ½ teaspoon sugar
- ⅛ teaspoon freshly ground black pepper

PER SERVING	2 thighs + about 1 cup veggies
CALORIES	429
FAT	20 g
SATURATED FAT	4 g
CHOLESTEROL	214 mg
CARBOHYDRATE	16 g
FIBER	4 g
PROTEIN	47 g
SUGAR	5 g
SODIUM	673 mg

CHICKEN AND VEGETABLES

8 (4-ounce) boneless, skinless chicken thighs, trimmed of fat

½ teaspoon kosher salt

12 ounces zucchini, cut into 1-inch cubes

3 carrots, cut into 1-inch cubes

1 red bell pepper, cut into 1-inch pieces

1 yellow bell pepper, cut into 1-inch pieces

1 red onion, chopped

Nonstick cooking spray

Chopped fresh parsley, for garnish

FOR THE MARINADE: In a large bowl, combine the oil, vinegar, garlic, salt, onion powder, oregano, basil, thyme, sugar, and black pepper.

FOR THE CHICKEN AND VEGETABLES: Season the chicken with the salt. Put the chicken, zucchini, carrots, bell peppers, and red onion in the bowl of marinade and toss well to coat. Marinate for 30 minutes or as long as overnight.

Arrange the oven racks in the center and lower third of the oven and preheat to 450°F. Coat two large nonstick rimmed baking sheets with cooking spray, or line with parchment paper or foil for easy cleanup.

Arrange the chicken and vegetables on the prepared baking sheets in a single layer. The vegetables and chicken should not touch.

Bake for 20 minutes. Flip the chicken and vegetables and bake until roasted and tender, 10 more minutes. Top with the parsley and serve.

Calories/Points Tracker

DATE ___/___/___ TO ___/___/___

	MONDAY			TUESDAY	
	FOODS	Calories/Points		FOODS	Calories/Points
BREAKFAST					
LUNCH					
DINNER					
SNACKS					
	DAILY TOTAL			DAILY TOTAL	

WEDNESDAY		THURSDAY	
FOODS	Calories/ Points	FOODS	Calories/ Points
DAILY TOTAL		DAILY TOTAL	

Calories/Points Tracker

DATE ____/____/____ TO ____/____/____

	FRIDAY			SATURDAY	
	FOODS	Calories/Points		FOODS	Calories/Points
BREAKFAST					
LUNCH					
DINNER					
SNACKS					
	DAILY TOTAL			DAILY TOTAL	

WEEKLY EXERCISE TRACKER

ACTIVITY

DISTANCE/DURATION/INTENSITY	CALORIES BURNED

SUNDAY	
FOODS	Calories/ Points
DAILY TOTAL	

TOTAL CALORIES BURNED	

MONDAY	−	=
TUESDAY	−	=
WEDNESDAY	−	=
THURSDAY	−	=
FRIDAY	−	=
SATURDAY	−	=
SUNDAY	−	=
WEEKLY CALORIES TOTALS	−	=
	Food	Exercise	Total

151

Weekly Meal Planner

DATE ___/___/___ TO ___/___/___

1. _____   M T W T F S S
   ☐ ☐ ☐ ☐ ☐ ☐ ☐

2. _____   M T W T F S S
   ☐ ☐ ☐ ☐ ☐ ☐ ☐

3. _____   M T W T F S S
   ☐ ☐ ☐ ☐ ☐ ☐ ☐

MONDAY	
B	
L	
D	

TUESDAY	
B	
L	
D	

WEDNESDAY	
B	
L	
D	

THURSDAY	
B	
L	
D	

FRIDAY	
B	
L	
D	

☐ _____

☐ _____

☐ _____

☐ _____

☐ _____

☐ _____

☐ _____

☐ _____

☐ _____

☐ _____

☐ _____

☐ _____

☐ _____

☐ _____

☐ _____

☐ _____

☐ _____

☐ _____

☐ _____

superfood WALNUTS

I love to toast walnuts to add to salads. Just put them on a baking sheet in a 350°F oven, stirring halfway through, until golden brown, about 10 minutes—and you're set!

NOTES

SATURDAY	
B	
L	
D	

SUNDAY	
B	
L	
D	

Calories/Points Tracker

DATE ___/___/___ TO ___/___/___

	MONDAY			TUESDAY	
	FOODS	Calories/Points		FOODS	Calories/Points
BREAKFAST					
LUNCH					
DINNER					
SNACKS					
	DAILY TOTAL			DAILY TOTAL	

WEDNESDAY		THURSDAY	
FOODS	Calories/Points	FOODS	Calories/Points
DAILY TOTAL		DAILY TOTAL	

Calories/Points Tracker

DATE ____ / ____ / ____ TO ____ / ____ / ____

	FRIDAY		SATURDAY	
	FOODS	Calories/Points	FOODS	Calories/Points
BREAKFAST				
LUNCH				
DINNER				
SNACKS				
	DAILY TOTAL		DAILY TOTAL	

WEEKLY EXERCISE TRACKER

ACTIVITY	
DISTANCE/DURATION/INTENSITY	CALORIES BURNED

SUNDAY	
FOODS	Calories/ Points
DAILY TOTAL	

TOTAL CALORIES BURNED	

	Food	Exercise	Total
MONDAY		-	=
TUESDAY		-	=
WEDNESDAY		-	=
THURSDAY		-	=
FRIDAY		-	=
SATURDAY		-	=
SUNDAY		-	=
WEEKLY CALORIES TOTALS		-	=

Weekly Meal Planner

DATE ___ / ___ / ___ TO ___ / ___ / ___

WEEKLY GOALS

1. _____
M T W T F S S
☐ ☐ ☐ ☐ ☐ ☐ ☐

2. _____
M T W T F S S
☐ ☐ ☐ ☐ ☐ ☐ ☐

3. _____
M T W T F S S
☐ ☐ ☐ ☐ ☐ ☐ ☐

MONDAY
B
L
D

TUESDAY
B
L
D

WEDNESDAY
B
L
D

THURSDAY
B
L
D

FRIDAY
B
L
D

SHOPPING LIST

- [ ] _____
- [ ] _____
- [ ] _____
- [ ] _____
- [ ] _____
- [ ] _____
- [ ] _____
- [ ] _____
- [ ] _____
- [ ] _____
- [ ] _____
- [ ] _____
- [ ] _____
- [ ] _____
- [ ] _____
- [ ] _____
- [ ] _____
- [ ] _____
- [ ] _____

"You can never cross the ocean until you have the courage to lose sight of the shore."

CHRISTOPHER COLUMBUS

NOTES

	SATURDAY
B	
L	
D	

	SUNDAY
B	
L	
D	

Calories/Points Tracker

DATE ___ / ___ / ___ TO ___ / ___ / ___

	MONDAY			TUESDAY	
	FOODS	Calories/Points		FOODS	Calories/Points
BREAKFAST					
LUNCH					
DINNER					
SNACKS					
	DAILY TOTAL			DAILY TOTAL	

WEDNESDAY		THURSDAY	
FOODS	Calories/ Points	FOODS	Calories/ Points
DAILY TOTAL		DAILY TOTAL	

Calories/Points Tracker

DATE ___ / ___ / ___ TO ___ / ___ / ___

	FRIDAY			SATURDAY	
	FOODS	Calories/Points		FOODS	Calories/Points
BREAKFAST					
LUNCH					
DINNER					
SNACKS					
	DAILY TOTAL			DAILY TOTAL	

162

WEEKLY EXERCISE TRACKER

SUNDAY	
FOODS	Calories/ Points
DAILY TOTAL	

ACTIVITY	
DISTANCE/DURATION/INTENSITY	CALORIES BURNED
TOTAL CALORIES BURNED	

MONDAY		-	=
TUESDAY		-	=
WEDNESDAY		-	=
THURSDAY		-	=
FRIDAY		-	=
SATURDAY		-	=
SUNDAY		-	=
WEEKLY CALORIES TOTALS	Food	Exercise	Total

Weekly Meal Planner

DATE ___ / ___ / ___ TO ___ / ___ / ___

WEEKLY GOALS

1. _____ M T W T F S S ☐ ☐ ☐ ☐ ☐ ☐ ☐

2. _____ M T W T F S S ☐ ☐ ☐ ☐ ☐ ☐ ☐

3. _____ M T W T F S S ☐ ☐ ☐ ☐ ☐ ☐ ☐

MONDAY	
B	
L	
D	

TUESDAY	
B	
L	
D	

WEDNESDAY	
B	
L	
D	

THURSDAY	
B	
L	
D	

FRIDAY	
B	
L	
D	

☐ _____
☐ _____
☐ _____
☐ _____
☐ _____
☐ _____
☐ _____
☐ _____
☐ _____
☐ _____
☐ _____
☐ _____
☐ _____
☐ _____
☐ _____
☐ _____
☐ _____
☐ _____
☐ _____

superfood BROCCOLI

Delicious cooked or raw, broccoli is wonderful added to pastas, frittatas and omelets, and salads, or eaten on its own.

NOTES

_____
_____
_____
_____
_____
_____
_____
_____
_____
_____
_____

SATURDAY	
B	
L	
D	

SUNDAY	
B	
L	
D	

Calories/Points Tracker

DATE ___ / ___ / ___ TO ___ / ___ / ___

	MONDAY			TUESDAY	
	FOODS	*Calories/ Points*		FOODS	*Calories/ Points*
BREAKFAST					
LUNCH					
DINNER					
SNACKS					
	DAILY TOTAL			DAILY TOTAL	

WEDNESDAY		THURSDAY	
FOODS	Calories/ Points	FOODS	Calories/ Points
DAILY TOTAL		DAILY TOTAL	

Calories/Points Tracker

DATE ___ / ___ / ___ TO ___ / ___ / ___

	FRIDAY			SATURDAY	
	FOODS	Calories/Points		FOODS	Calories/Points
BREAKFAST					
LUNCH					
DINNER					
SNACKS					
	DAILY TOTAL			DAILY TOTAL	

WEEKLY EXERCISE TRACKER

SUNDAY	
FOODS	Calories/ Points
DAILY TOTAL	

ACTIVITY

DISTANCE/DURATION/INTENSITY	CALORIES BURNED
TOTAL CALORIES BURNED	

MONDAY		–	=
TUESDAY		–	=
WEDNESDAY		–	=
THURSDAY		–	=
FRIDAY		–	=
SATURDAY		–	=
SUNDAY		–	=
WEEKLY CALORIES TOTALS	Food	Exercise	Total

Whole Wheat Linguine with Spicy Sausage and Roasted Peppers

I love everything about this meal, especially that it's ready in under 30 minutes! I like using spicy chicken sausage to give it a little kick, but if you want to make this mild for your family, simply swap it for sweet Italian.

SERVES ABOUT 4

14 ounces hot Italian chicken sausage

1 teaspoon olive oil

1 (12-ounce) jar water-packed roasted red peppers, drained and chopped

⅓ cup chopped onion

3 garlic cloves, crushed with the side of a knife

Kosher salt and freshly ground black pepper

1½ cups canned crushed tomatoes

½ cup low-sodium chicken broth

9 ounces whole wheat (or gluten-free) linguine (I like DeLallo)

2 tablespoons freshly grated Pecorino Romano cheese

1 tablespoon chopped fresh parsley

PER SERVING	1½ cups
CALORIES	372
FAT	11 g
SATURATED FAT	2.5 g
CHOLESTEROL	67 mg
CARBOHYDRATE	49 g
FIBER	5.5 g
PROTEIN	21 g
SUGAR	7 g
SODIUM	911 mg (without added salt)

In a large skillet set over medium heat, cook the sausage, using a wooden spoon to break the meat into pieces as it browns, 4 to 5 minutes. Transfer the sausage to a plate.

To the skillet, add the oil, roasted peppers, onion, garlic, and salt and black pepper to taste. Cook, stirring, until soft, 4 to 5 minutes. Add the tomatoes and broth and return the sausage to the skillet. Bring to a boil, reduce the heat to low, and simmer for 15 minutes.

Meanwhile, in a large pot of salted boiling water, cook the pasta to al dente according to the package directions.

Drain the pasta and toss into the pan of sauce. Add the pecorino, toss well, and cook, stirring, to marry the flavors, about 2 minutes. Sprinkle with the parsley and serve.

Weekly Meal Planner

DATE ___ / ___ / ___ TO ___ / ___ / ___

WEEKLY GOALS

1. _____ M T W T F S S ☐☐☐☐☐☐☐

2. _____ M T W T F S S ☐☐☐☐☐☐☐

3. _____ M T W T F S S ☐☐☐☐☐☐☐

MONDAY	
B	
L	
D	

TUESDAY	
B	
L	
D	

WEDNESDAY	
B	
L	
D	

THURSDAY	
B	
L	
D	

FRIDAY	
B	
L	
D	

SHOPPING LIST

- [ ] _____
- [ ] _____
- [ ] _____
- [ ] _____
- [ ] _____
- [ ] _____
- [ ] _____
- [ ] _____
- [ ] _____
- [ ] _____
- [ ] _____
- [ ] _____
- [ ] _____
- [ ] _____
- [ ] _____
- [ ] _____
- [ ] _____
- [ ] _____
- [ ] _____

> "Life shrinks or expands in proportion to one's courage."
>
> ANAïS NIN

NOTES

SATURDAY	
B	
L	
D	

SUNDAY	
B	
L	
D	

Calories/Points Tracker

DATE ___ / ___ / ___ TO ___ / ___ / ___

	MONDAY			TUESDAY	
	FOODS	Calories/Points		FOODS	Calories/Points
BREAKFAST					
LUNCH					
DINNER					
SNACKS					
	DAILY TOTAL			DAILY TOTAL	

WEDNESDAY		THURSDAY	
FOODS	Calories/ Points	FOODS	Calories/ Points
DAILY TOTAL		DAILY TOTAL	

Calories/Points Tracker

DATE ___ / ___ / ___ TO ___ / ___ / ___

	FRIDAY			SATURDAY	
	FOODS	Calories/Points		FOODS	Calories/Points
BREAKFAST					
LUNCH					
DINNER					
SNACKS					
	DAILY TOTAL			DAILY TOTAL	

WEEKLY EXERCISE TRACKER

SUNDAY	
FOODS	Calories/ Points
DAILY TOTAL	

ACTIVITY	
DISTANCE/DURATION/INTENSITY	CALORIES BURNED
TOTAL CALORIES BURNED	

MONDAY		-	=
TUESDAY		-	=
WEDNESDAY		-	=
THURSDAY		-	=
FRIDAY		-	=
SATURDAY		-	=
SUNDAY		-	=
WEEKLY CALORIES TOTALS		-	=
	Food	Exercise	Total

Weekly Meal Planner

DATE ___ / ___ / ___ TO ___ / ___ / ___

WEEKLY GOALS

1. _____ M T W T F S S
   ☐ ☐ ☐ ☐ ☐ ☐ ☐

2. _____ M T W T F S S
   ☐ ☐ ☐ ☐ ☐ ☐ ☐

3. _____ M T W T F S S
   ☐ ☐ ☐ ☐ ☐ ☐ ☐

MONDAY

B	
L	
D	

TUESDAY

B	
L	
D	

WEDNESDAY

B	
L	
D	

THURSDAY

B	
L	
D	

FRIDAY

B	
L	
D	

SHOPPING LIST

- [ ] _____
- [ ] _____
- [ ] _____
- [ ] _____
- [ ] _____
- [ ] _____
- [ ] _____
- [ ] _____
- [ ] _____
- [ ] _____
- [ ] _____
- [ ] _____
- [ ] _____
- [ ] _____
- [ ] _____
- [ ] _____
- [ ] _____
- [ ] _____
- [ ] _____
- [ ] _____

> "Go confidently in the direction of your dreams. Live the life you have imagined."
>
> HENRY DAVID THOREAU

NOTES

_____
_____
_____
_____
_____
_____
_____
_____
_____
_____
_____
_____
_____

SATURDAY	
B	
L	
D	

SUNDAY	
B	
L	
D	

Calories/Points Tracker

DATE ____ / ____ / ____ TO ____ / ____ / ____

	MONDAY			TUESDAY	
	FOODS	Calories/Points		FOODS	Calories/Points
BREAKFAST					
LUNCH					
DINNER					
SNACKS					
	DAILY TOTAL			DAILY TOTAL	

WEDNESDAY		THURSDAY	
FOODS	Calories/Points	FOODS	Calories/Points
DAILY TOTAL		DAILY TOTAL	

Calories/Points Tracker

DATE ___ / ___ / ___ TO ___ / ___ / ___

	FRIDAY			SATURDAY	
	FOODS	Calories/Points		FOODS	Calories/Points
BREAKFAST					
LUNCH					
DINNER					
SNACKS					
	DAILY TOTAL			DAILY TOTAL	

WEEKLY EXERCISE TRACKER

ACTIVITY	
DISTANCE/DURATION/INTENSITY	CALORIES BURNED

SUNDAY	
FOODS	Calories/ Points
DAILY TOTAL	

TOTAL CALORIES BURNED

MONDAY	–	=
TUESDAY	–	=
WEDNESDAY	–	=
THURSDAY	–	=
FRIDAY	–	=
SATURDAY	–	=
SUNDAY	–	=
WEEKLY CALORIES TOTALS	–	=
	Food	Exercise	Total

Weekly Meal Planner

DATE ____ / ____ / ____ TO ____ / ____ / ____

WEEKLY GOALS

1. _____ M T W T F S S ☐☐☐☐☐☐☐

2. _____ M T W T F S S ☐☐☐☐☐☐☐

3. _____ M T W T F S S ☐☐☐☐☐☐☐

MONDAY	
B	
L	
D	

TUESDAY	
B	
L	
D	

WEDNESDAY	
B	
L	
D	

THURSDAY	
B	
L	
D	

FRIDAY	
B	
L	
D	

SHOPPING LIST

- [ ] _____
- [ ] _____
- [ ] _____
- [ ] _____
- [ ] _____
- [ ] _____
- [ ] _____
- [ ] _____
- [ ] _____
- [ ] _____
- [ ] _____
- [ ] _____
- [ ] _____
- [ ] _____
- [ ] _____
- [ ] _____
- [ ] _____
- [ ] _____
- [ ] _____

superfood SALMON

Salmon is really easy to prepare—trust me! And leftovers are delicious the next day served chilled and with a salad.

NOTES

SATURDAY	
B	
L	
D	

SUNDAY	
B	
L	
D	

Calories/Points Tracker

DATE ___ / ___ / ___ TO ___ / ___ / ___

	MONDAY			TUESDAY	
	FOODS	Calories/Points		FOODS	Calories/Points
BREAKFAST					
LUNCH					
DINNER					
SNACKS					
	DAILY TOTAL			DAILY TOTAL	

WEDNESDAY		THURSDAY	
FOODS	Calories/ Points	FOODS	Calories/ Points
DAILY TOTAL		DAILY TOTAL	

Calories/Points Tracker

DATE _____ / ___ / ___ TO _____ / ___ / ___

	FRIDAY			SATURDAY	
	FOODS	Calories/ Points		FOODS	Calories/ Points
BREAKFAST					
LUNCH					
DINNER					
SNACKS					
	DAILY TOTAL			DAILY TOTAL	

WEEKLY EXERCISE TRACKER

SUNDAY	
FOODS	Calories/ Points
DAILY TOTAL	

ACTIVITY	
DISTANCE/DURATION/INTENSITY	CALORIES BURNED

TOTAL CALORIES BURNED	

MONDAY	−	=
TUESDAY	−	=
WEDNESDAY	−	=
THURSDAY	−	=
FRIDAY	−	=
SATURDAY	−	=
SUNDAY	−	=
WEEKLY CALORIES TOTALS	−	=
	Food	Exercise	Total

Weekly Meal Planner

DATE ____ / ____ / ____ TO ____ / ____ / ____

WEEKLY GOALS

1. _____ M T W T F S S
   ☐ ☐ ☐ ☐ ☐ ☐ ☐

2. _____ M T W T F S S
   ☐ ☐ ☐ ☐ ☐ ☐ ☐

3. _____ M T W T F S S
   ☐ ☐ ☐ ☐ ☐ ☐ ☐

MONDAY
B
L
D

TUESDAY
B
L
D

WEDNESDAY
B
L
D

THURSDAY
B
L
D

FRIDAY
B
L
D

SHOPPING LIST

- [ ] _____
- [ ] _____
- [ ] _____
- [ ] _____
- [ ] _____
- [ ] _____
- [ ] _____
- [ ] _____
- [ ] _____
- [ ] _____
- [ ] _____
- [ ] _____
- [ ] _____
- [ ] _____
- [ ] _____
- [ ] _____
- [ ] _____
- [ ] _____
- [ ] _____
- [ ] _____

> "Start where you are.
> Use what you have.
> Do what you can."
>
> ARTHUR ASHE

NOTES

_____
_____
_____
_____
_____
_____
_____
_____
_____
_____
_____

SATURDAY	
B	
L	
D	

SUNDAY	
B	
L	
D	

Calories/Points Tracker

DATE ___ / ___ / ___ TO ___ / ___ / ___

	MONDAY			TUESDAY	
	FOODS	Calories/Points		FOODS	Calories/Points
BREAKFAST					
LUNCH					
DINNER					
SNACKS					
	DAILY TOTAL			DAILY TOTAL	

WEDNESDAY		THURSDAY	
FOODS	Calories/ Points	FOODS	Calories/ Points
DAILY TOTAL		DAILY TOTAL	

Chicken and Andouille Sausage

On Fat Tuesday one year, I had gumbo on my mind. The traditional Cajun dish has lots of fat, and it takes a long time to make, so I came up with this recipe in an effort to lighten it up some and satisfy my craving quick. This is the type of dish you may want to eat with a fork and a spoon! I served mine with ¼ cup of cooked brown rice on the side, which is optional. Quinoa or farro would also work nicely.

SERVES 4

- 2 teaspoons olive oil
- 1 cup chopped onion
- ½ cup chopped green bell pepper
- ¼ cup chopped celery
- 4 (5-ounce) bone-in, skinless chicken thighs, trimmed of fat
- 4 (3-ounce) bone-in, skinless chicken drumsticks, trimmed of fat
- 1 teaspoon kosher salt
- Freshly ground black pepper
- 1 tablespoon all-purpose flour (or rice flour for gluten-free)
- 2 (3-ounce) links fully cooked chicken/turkey andouille sausage, sliced ½ inch thick (I like Applegate)
- 1 bay leaf
- ¼ cup chopped scallions

PER SERVING	1 drumstick, 1 thigh + 1.5 ounces sausage + broth
CALORIES	319.5
FAT	12 g
SATURATED FAT	3 g
CHOLESTEROL	194.5 mg
CARBOHYDRATE	8 g
FIBER	1.5 g
PROTEIN	42.5 g
SUGAR	1 g
SODIUM	744 mg

Heat a large, deep nonstick skillet over medium heat. When hot, add the oil, onion, bell pepper, and celery. Cook, stirring, until soft, 3 to 4 minutes. Push the vegetables to the edges of the skillet and add the chicken. Season the chicken with the salt and black pepper to taste and cook until browned, 2 to 3 minutes per side. Sprinkle the flour over the chicken and vegetables. Add 2 cups water, the sausage, and bay leaf, then cover and reduce the heat to low. Simmer for 30 to 35 minutes. Remove the bay leaf. Serve topped with the scallions.

Tomato Tuna Melts

I swapped the bread for tomatoes in these quick and easy low-carb tuna melts made with tuna salad and melted cheddar. They're wonderful for lunch and a great way to use up summer tomatoes. Best of all, they only take 5 minutes to make!

SERVES 2

2 tomatoes, cut in half horizontally

2 pinches of kosher salt

   Freshly ground black pepper

1 (5-ounce) can water-packed solid white tuna, slightly drained

3 tablespoons finely chopped celery

1 tablespoon finely chopped red onion

2 tablespoons light mayonnaise

1 teaspoon red wine vinegar

4 slices cheddar cheese (2½ ounces total)

PER SERVING	2 halves
CALORIES	267
FAT	16 g
SATURATED FAT	8.5 g
CHOLESTEROL	67 mg
CARBOHYDRATE	8 g
FIBER	1.5 g
PROTEIN	24 g
SUGAR	0 g
SODIUM	611 mg

Adjust an oven rack about 4 inches from the flame and preheat the broiler to high.

Arrange the tomatoes on a baking sheet cut sides up and season with the salt and pepper to taste.

In a small bowl, combine the tuna, celery, red onion, mayonnaise, and vinegar. Spoon ¼ cup of the tuna salad onto each tomato half and top with a slice of cheese.

Broil until the cheese is melted, 1 to 2 minutes. Serve immediately.

Calories/Points Tracker

DATE _____ / ___ / _____ TO _____ / ___ / _____

	FRIDAY			SATURDAY	
	FOODS	Calories/Points		FOODS	Calories/Points
BREAKFAST					
LUNCH					
DINNER					
SNACKS					
	DAILY TOTAL			DAILY TOTAL	

WEEKLY EXERCISE TRACKER

ACTIVITY	
DISTANCE/DURATION/INTENSITY	CALORIES BURNED

TOTAL CALORIES BURNED	

SUNDAY

FOODS	Calories/ Points
DAILY TOTAL	

MONDAY		–	=
TUESDAY		–	=
WEDNESDAY		–	=
THURSDAY		–	=
FRIDAY		–	=
SATURDAY		–	=
SUNDAY		–	=
WEEKLY CALORIES TOTALS		–	=
	Food	Exercise	Total

Weekly Meal Planner

DATE _____ / _____ / _____ TO _____ / _____ / _____

WEEKLY GOALS

1. _____
   M T W T F S S
   ☐ ☐ ☐ ☐ ☐ ☐ ☐

2. _____
   M T W T F S S
   ☐ ☐ ☐ ☐ ☐ ☐ ☐

3. _____
   M T W T F S S
   ☐ ☐ ☐ ☐ ☐ ☐ ☐

MONDAY
B
L
D

TUESDAY
B
L
D

WEDNESDAY
B
L
D

THURSDAY
B
L
D

FRIDAY
B
L
D

- [ ] _____
- [ ] _____
- [ ] _____
- [ ] _____
- [ ] _____
- [ ] _____
- [ ] _____
- [ ] _____
- [ ] _____
- [ ] _____
- [ ] _____
- [ ] _____
- [ ] _____
- [ ] _____
- [ ] _____
- [ ] _____
- [ ] _____
- [ ] _____
- [ ] _____

superfood YOGURT

Yogurt is one of the quickest breakfasts you can eat, and you can mix in other healthy foods like berries and fruit, granola, or a little honey.

NOTES

SATURDAY	
B	
L	
D	

SUNDAY	
B	
L	
D	

Calories/Points Tracker

DATE ___ / ___ / ___ TO ___ / ___ / ___

	MONDAY			TUESDAY	
	FOODS	Calories/ Points		FOODS	Calories/ Points
BREAKFAST					
LUNCH					
DINNER					
SNACKS					
	DAILY TOTAL			DAILY TOTAL	

WEDNESDAY			THURSDAY	
FOODS	Calories/ Points		FOODS	Calories/ Points
DAILY TOTAL			DAILY TOTAL	

Calories/Points Tracker

DATE ____ / ____ / ____ TO ____ / ____ / ____

	FRIDAY			SATURDAY	
	FOODS	Calories/Points		FOODS	Calories/Points
BREAKFAST					
LUNCH					
DINNER					
SNACKS					
	DAILY TOTAL			DAILY TOTAL	

DAILY CALORIES/
POINTS GOALS

WEEKLY EXERCISE TRACKER

SUNDAY	
FOODS	*Calories/ Points*
DAILY TOTAL	

ACTIVITY	
DISTANCE/DURATION/INTENSITY	CALORIES BURNED
TOTAL CALORIES BURNED	

MONDAY	-	=	
TUESDAY	-	=	
WEDNESDAY	-	=	
THURSDAY	-	=	
FRIDAY	-	=	
SATURDAY	-	=	
SUNDAY	-	=	
WEEKLY CALORIES TOTALS	-	=	
	Food	*Exercise*	*Total*

Weekly Meal Planner

DATE ____/____/____ TO ____/____/____

WEEKLY GOALS

1. _____ M T W T F S S
   ☐☐☐☐☐☐☐

2. _____ M T W T F S S
   ☐☐☐☐☐☐☐

3. _____ M T W T F S S
   ☐☐☐☐☐☐☐

MONDAY	
B	
L	
D	

TUESDAY	
B	
L	
D	

WEDNESDAY	
B	
L	
D	

THURSDAY	
B	
L	
D	

FRIDAY	
B	
L	
D	

SHOPPING LIST

- [ ] _____
- [ ] _____
- [ ] _____
- [ ] _____
- [ ] _____
- [ ] _____
- [ ] _____
- [ ] _____
- [ ] _____
- [ ] _____
- [ ] _____
- [ ] _____
- [ ] _____
- [ ] _____
- [ ] _____
- [ ] _____
- [ ] _____
- [ ] _____
- [ ] _____

> "Challenges are what make life interesting; overcoming them is what makes life meaningful."
>
> JOSHUA J. MARINE

NOTES

SATURDAY	
B	
L	
D	

SUNDAY	
B	
L	
D	

Calories/Points Tracker

DATE ___ / ___ / ___ TO ___ / ___ / ___

	MONDAY			TUESDAY	
	FOODS	Calories/Points		FOODS	Calories/Points
BREAKFAST					
LUNCH					
DINNER					
SNACKS					
	DAILY TOTAL			DAILY TOTAL	

WEDNESDAY		THURSDAY	
FOODS	Calories/ Points	FOODS	Calories/ Points
DAILY TOTAL		DAILY TOTAL	

Calories/Points Tracker

DATE ___ / ___ / ___ TO ___ / ___ / ___

	FRIDAY			SATURDAY	
	FOODS	Calories/Points		FOODS	Calories/Points
BREAKFAST					
LUNCH					
DINNER					
SNACKS					
	DAILY TOTAL			DAILY TOTAL	

WEEKLY EXERCISE TRACKER

SUNDAY	
FOODS	Calories/ Points
DAILY TOTAL	

ACTIVITY	
DISTANCE/DURATION/INTENSITY	CALORIES BURNED
TOTAL CALORIES BURNED	

MONDAY	-	=	
TUESDAY	-	=	
WEDNESDAY	-	=	
THURSDAY	-	=	
FRIDAY	-	=	
SATURDAY	-	=	
SUNDAY	-	=	
WEEKLY CALORIES TOTALS	-	=	
	Food	Exercise	Total

Weekly Meal Planner

DATE ___ / ___ / ___ TO ___ / ___ / ___

WEEKLY GOALS

1. _____ M T W T F S S
   ☐ ☐ ☐ ☐ ☐ ☐ ☐

2. _____ M T W T F S S
   ☐ ☐ ☐ ☐ ☐ ☐ ☐

3. _____ M T W T F S S
   ☐ ☐ ☐ ☐ ☐ ☐ ☐

MONDAY
B
L
D

TUESDAY
B
L
D

WEDNESDAY
B
L
D

THURSDAY
B
L
D

FRIDAY
B
L
D

SHOPPING LIST

☐ _____
☐ _____
☐ _____
☐ _____
☐ _____
☐ _____
☐ _____
☐ _____
☐ _____
☐ _____
☐ _____
☐ _____
☐ _____
☐ _____
☐ _____
☐ _____
☐ _____
☐ _____
☐ _____

"If you want to lift yourself up, lift up someone else."

BOOKER T. WASHINGTON

NOTES

_____
_____
_____
_____
_____
_____
_____
_____
_____

SATURDAY	
B	
L	
D	

SUNDAY	
B	
L	
D	

Calories/Points Tracker

DATE ___ / ___ / ___ TO ___ / ___ / ___

	MONDAY			TUESDAY	
	FOODS	Calories/Points		FOODS	Calories/Points
BREAKFAST					
LUNCH					
DINNER					
SNACKS					
	DAILY TOTAL			DAILY TOTAL	

WEDNESDAY		THURSDAY	
FOODS	Calories/ Points	FOODS	Calories/ Points
DAILY TOTAL		DAILY TOTAL	

Calories/Points Tracker

DATE ___ / ___ / ___ TO ___ / ___ / ___

	FRIDAY			SATURDAY	
	FOODS	Calories/ Points		FOODS	Calories/ Points
BREAKFAST					
LUNCH					
DINNER					
SNACKS					
	DAILY TOTAL			DAILY TOTAL	

WEEKLY EXERCISE TRACKER

SUNDAY	
FOODS	Calories/Points
DAILY TOTAL	

ACTIVITY	
DISTANCE/DURATION/INTENSITY	CALORIES BURNED
TOTAL CALORIES BURNED	

MONDAY	-	=
TUESDAY	-	=
WEDNESDAY	-	=
THURSDAY	-	=
FRIDAY	-	=
SATURDAY	-	=
SUNDAY	-	=
WEEKLY CALORIES TOTALS	-	=
	Food	Exercise	Total

Weekly Meal Planner

DATE ___/___/___ TO ___/___/___

WEEKLY GOALS

1. _____ M T W T F S S
   ☐ ☐ ☐ ☐ ☐ ☐ ☐

2. _____ M T W T F S S
   ☐ ☐ ☐ ☐ ☐ ☐ ☐

3. _____ M T W T F S S
   ☐ ☐ ☐ ☐ ☐ ☐ ☐

MONDAY	
B	
L	
D	

TUESDAY	
B	
L	
D	

WEDNESDAY	
B	
L	
D	

THURSDAY	
B	
L	
D	

FRIDAY	
B	
L	
D	

SHOPPING LIST

☐ _____
☐ _____
☐ _____
☐ _____
☐ _____
☐ _____
☐ _____
☐ _____
☐ _____
☐ _____
☐ _____
☐ _____
☐ _____
☐ _____
☐ _____
☐ _____
☐ _____
☐ _____
☐ _____

superfood KALE

You can do more with kale than make a salad! Try sautéing it with garlic for a side dish or adding it to frittatas and omelets.

NOTES

_____
_____
_____
_____
_____
_____
_____
_____
_____
_____
_____

SATURDAY	
B	
L	
D	

SUNDAY	
B	
L	
D	

Summer Corn, Tomato, and Avocado Salad with Creamy Buttermilk-Dijon Dressing

Take advantage of the end of summer's abundance of sweet corn and delicious ripe tomatoes with this easy side dish. It is perfect to go along with anything you're grilling and is a stunner at potluck parties. The dressing is creamy yet light, with just a touch of tang from the buttermilk.

SERVES 4

DRESSING

- 6 tablespoons 1% buttermilk
- 2 tablespoons extra-virgin olive oil
- 2 tablespoons white wine vinegar
- 2 teaspoons Dijon mustard
- 1 tablespoon minced shallot
- ¼ teaspoon garlic powder
- ½ teaspoon kosher salt
- Freshly ground black pepper

SALAD

- 1 medium ear corn
- 1 head romaine lettuce, chopped (about 5 cups)
- 4 or 5 large grape tomatoes, quartered
- 3 ounces sliced avocado (½ large Hass)
- ¼ cup sliced red onion

PER SERVING	1½ cups
CALORIES	147
FAT	11 g
SATURATED FAT	1.5 g
CHOLESTEROL	1 mg
CARBOHYDRATE	12 g
FIBER	3.5 g
PROTEIN	4 g
SUGAR	3 g
SODIUM	237 mg

FOR THE DRESSING: In a small bowl, whisk together the buttermilk, oil, vinegar, mustard, shallot, garlic powder, salt, and black pepper to taste.

FOR THE SALAD: First, cook the corn. The quickest way to do this is to microwave the corn, husk on, for 3 minutes. Let cool, peel off and discard the husk, then cut the kernels off the cob.

Place the lettuce in a large bowl. Top with the corn, tomatoes, avocado, and red onion. Drizzle with the dressing and serve.

Calories/Points Tracker

DATE ____ / ____ / ____ TO ____ / ____ / ____

	MONDAY			TUESDAY	
	FOODS	Calories/ Points		FOODS	Calories/ Points
BREAKFAST					
LUNCH					
DINNER					
SNACKS					
	DAILY TOTAL			DAILY TOTAL	

WEDNESDAY			THURSDAY	
FOODS	Calories/ Points		FOODS	Calories/ Points
DAILY TOTAL			DAILY TOTAL	

Calories/Points Tracker

DATE ___ / ___ / ___ TO ___ / ___ / ___

	FRIDAY			SATURDAY	
	FOODS	Calories/ Points		FOODS	Calories/ Points
BREAKFAST					
LUNCH					
DINNER					
SNACKS					
	DAILY TOTAL			DAILY TOTAL	

WEEKLY EXERCISE TRACKER

ACTIVITY	
DISTANCE/DURATION/INTENSITY	CALORIES BURNED

SUNDAY	
FOODS	Calories/ Points
DAILY TOTAL	

TOTAL CALORIES BURNED	

MONDAY	–	=	
TUESDAY	–	=	
WEDNESDAY	–	=	
THURSDAY	–	=	
FRIDAY	–	=	
SATURDAY	–	=	
SUNDAY	–	=	
WEEKLY CALORIES TOTALS	–	=	
	Food	Exercise	Total

Weekly Meal Planner

DATE _____ / _____ / _____ TO _____ / _____ / _____

WEEKLY GOALS

1. _____ M T W T F S S
   ☐ ☐ ☐ ☐ ☐ ☐ ☐

2. _____ M T W T F S S
   ☐ ☐ ☐ ☐ ☐ ☐ ☐

3. _____ M T W T F S S
   ☐ ☐ ☐ ☐ ☐ ☐ ☐

MONDAY
B
L
D

TUESDAY
B
L
D

WEDNESDAY
B
L
D

THURSDAY
B
L
D

FRIDAY
B
L
D

SHOPPING LIST

- [ ] _____
- [ ] _____
- [ ] _____
- [ ] _____
- [ ] _____
- [ ] _____
- [ ] _____
- [ ] _____
- [ ] _____
- [ ] _____
- [ ] _____
- [ ] _____
- [ ] _____
- [ ] _____
- [ ] _____
- [ ] _____
- [ ] _____
- [ ] _____
- [ ] _____

> "Limitations live only in our minds."
>
> JAMIE PAOLINETTI

NOTES

	SATURDAY
B	
L	
D	

	SUNDAY
B	
L	
D	

Calories/Points Tracker

DATE ____ / ____ / ____ TO ____ / ____ / ____

	MONDAY			TUESDAY	
	FOODS	Calories/ Points		FOODS	Calories/ Points
BREAKFAST					
LUNCH					
DINNER					
SNACKS					
	DAILY TOTAL			DAILY TOTAL	

226

WEDNESDAY		THURSDAY	
FOODS	Calories/Points	FOODS	Calories/Points
DAILY TOTAL		DAILY TOTAL	

Calories/Points Tracker

DATE ___ / ___ / ___ TO ___ / ___ / ___

FRIDAY		SATURDAY	
FOODS	Calories/Points	FOODS	Calories/Points
BREAKFAST			
LUNCH			
DINNER			
SNACKS			
DAILY TOTAL		DAILY TOTAL	

WEEKLY EXERCISE TRACKER

SUNDAY	
FOODS	Calories/ Points
DAILY TOTAL	

ACTIVITY		
DISTANCE/DURATION/INTENSITY		CALORIES BURNED
TOTAL CALORIES BURNED		

MONDAY		-	=
TUESDAY		-	=
WEDNESDAY		-	=
THURSDAY		-	=
FRIDAY		-	=
SATURDAY		-	=
SUNDAY		-	=
WEEKLY CALORIES TOTALS		-	=
	Food	Exercise	Total

Weekly Meal Planner

DATE ___ / ___ / ___ TO ___ / ___ / ___

WEEKLY GOALS

1. _____ M T W T F S S
   ☐ ☐ ☐ ☐ ☐ ☐ ☐

2. _____ M T W T F S S
   ☐ ☐ ☐ ☐ ☐ ☐ ☐

3. _____ M T W T F S S
   ☐ ☐ ☐ ☐ ☐ ☐ ☐

MONDAY	
B	
L	
D	

TUESDAY	
B	
L	
D	

WEDNESDAY	
B	
L	
D	

THURSDAY	
B	
L	
D	

FRIDAY	
B	
L	
D	

SHOPPING LIST

- [ ] _____
- [ ] _____
- [ ] _____
- [ ] _____
- [ ] _____
- [ ] _____
- [ ] _____
- [ ] _____
- [ ] _____
- [ ] _____
- [ ] _____
- [ ] _____
- [ ] _____
- [ ] _____
- [ ] _____
- [ ] _____
- [ ] _____
- [ ] _____
- [ ] _____
- [ ] _____

superfood APPLES

An apple a day . . . keeps you healthy, always! Apples are a perfectly compact, portable snack, as well as a delicious add-in to salads.

NOTES

SATURDAY	
B	
L	
D	

SUNDAY	
B	
L	
D	

Calories/Points Tracker

	MONDAY			TUESDAY	
	FOODS	Calories/ Points		FOODS	Calories/ Points
BREAKFAST					
LUNCH					
DINNER					
SNACKS					
	DAILY TOTAL			DAILY TOTAL	

DAILY CALORIES/
POINTS GOALS

WEDNESDAY	
FOODS	Calories/Points
DAILY TOTAL	

THURSDAY	
FOODS	Calories/Points
DAILY TOTAL	

Calories/Points Tracker

DATE ___ / ___ / ___ TO ___ / ___ / ___

	FRIDAY			SATURDAY	
	FOODS	Calories/ Points		FOODS	Calories/ Points
BREAKFAST					
LUNCH					
DINNER					
SNACKS					
	DAILY TOTAL			DAILY TOTAL	

WEEKLY EXERCISE TRACKER

SUNDAY	
FOODS	Calories/ Points
DAILY TOTAL	

ACTIVITY	
DISTANCE/DURATION/INTENSITY	CALORIES BURNED
TOTAL CALORIES BURNED	

MONDAY	-	=	
TUESDAY	-	=	
WEDNESDAY	-	=	
THURSDAY	-	=	
FRIDAY	-	=	
SATURDAY	-	=	
SUNDAY	-	=	
WEEKLY CALORIES TOTALS	-	=	
	Food	Exercise	Total

Weekly Meal Planner

DATE ____ / ____ / ____ TO ____ / ____ / ____

WEEKLY GOALS

M T W T F S S

1. _____ ☐☐☐☐☐☐☐

M T W T F S S

2. _____ ☐☐☐☐☐☐☐

M T W T F S S

3. _____ ☐☐☐☐☐☐☐

MONDAY	
B	
L	
D	

TUESDAY	
B	
L	
D	

WEDNESDAY	
B	
L	
D	

THURSDAY	
B	
L	
D	

FRIDAY	
B	
L	
D	

- [ ] _____
- [ ] _____
- [ ] _____
- [ ] _____
- [ ] _____
- [ ] _____
- [ ] _____
- [ ] _____
- [ ] _____
- [ ] _____
- [ ] _____
- [ ] _____
- [ ] _____
- [ ] _____
- [ ] _____
- [ ] _____
- [ ] _____
- [ ] _____
- [ ] _____
- [ ] _____

> "It is never too late to be what you might have been."
>
> GEORGE ELIOT

NOTES

_____
_____
_____
_____
_____
_____
_____
_____
_____
_____
_____
_____

SATURDAY	
B	
L	
D	

SUNDAY	
B	
L	
D	

Calories/Points Tracker

DATE ___ / ___ / ___ TO ___ / ___ / ___

	MONDAY			TUESDAY	
	FOODS	Calories/ Points		FOODS	Calories/ Points
BREAKFAST					
LUNCH					
DINNER					
SNACKS					
	DAILY TOTAL			DAILY TOTAL	

WEDNESDAY			THURSDAY	
FOODS	Calories/ Points		FOODS	Calories/ Points
DAILY TOTAL			DAILY TOTAL	

Calories/Points Tracker

DATE ___/___/___ TO ___/___/___

	FRIDAY			SATURDAY	
	FOODS	Calories/Points		FOODS	Calories/Points
BREAKFAST					
LUNCH					
DINNER					
SNACKS					
	DAILY TOTAL			DAILY TOTAL	

WEEKLY EXERCISE TRACKER

ACTIVITY	
DISTANCE/DURATION/INTENSITY	CALORIES BURNED

SUNDAY	
FOODS	Calories/ Points
DAILY TOTAL	

TOTAL CALORIES BURNED	

MONDAY	– =
TUESDAY	– =
WEDNESDAY	– =
THURSDAY	– =
FRIDAY	– =
SATURDAY	– =
SUNDAY	– =
WEEKLY CALORIES TOTALS	– =
	Food Exercise Total

Grilled Flank Steak with Black Beans, Corn, and Tomatoes

This steak dish is a fiesta of flavors! I love topping grilled meats with fresh salad. In this Tex-Mex version, you can easily tweak the flavors to suit your family's taste—make it spicy with some chopped jalapeños, or swap out an ingredient for those picky kids.

SERVES 6

1½ pounds flank steak

2 garlic cloves, crushed with the side of a knife

½ teaspoon ground cumin

¾ teaspoon kosher salt

Freshly ground black pepper

3 tablespoons minced red onion

1 teaspoon olive oil

¼ cup fresh lime juice

2 medium vine tomatoes, chopped

1 cup canned black beans, rinsed and drained

1 cup frozen or fresh corn kernels

2 tablespoons finely chopped fresh cilantro

Olive oil or olive oil spray, for greasing

PER SERVING	3 ounces steak + ¾ cup salad
CALORIES	248
FAT	9.5 g
SATURATED FAT	3.5 g
CHOLESTEROL	57 mg
CARBOHYDRATE	15 g
FIBER	3 g
PROTEIN	27 g
SUGAR	3 g
SODIUM	378 mg

Rub the steak all over with the crushed garlic, cumin, ½ teaspoon of the salt, and pepper to taste. Let sit for 5 to 10 minutes.

In a medium bowl, combine the red onion, olive oil, lime juice, remaining ¼ teaspoon salt, and pepper to taste. Let sit for 5 minutes. Add the tomatoes, black beans, corn, and cilantro and stir well.

Preheat a grill to high heat (or preheat a grill pan over high heat). When hot, rub the grates with oil (or spray the pan with oil). Grill the steak to your desired doneness; 6 to 8 minutes will be medium. Transfer the steak to a cutting board and let it rest for 5 minutes before slicing.

Thinly slice the beef across the grain, place it on a platter, and top with the corn salad. Serve.

Weekly Meal Planner

DATE ___ / ___ / ___ TO ___ / ___ / ___

WEEKLY GOALS

1. _____ M T W T F S S
   ☐ ☐ ☐ ☐ ☐ ☐ ☐

2. _____ M T W T F S S
   ☐ ☐ ☐ ☐ ☐ ☐ ☐

3. _____ M T W T F S S
   ☐ ☐ ☐ ☐ ☐ ☐ ☐

MONDAY

B	
L	
D	

TUESDAY

B	
L	
D	

WEDNESDAY

B	
L	
D	

THURSDAY

B	
L	
D	

FRIDAY

B	
L	
D	

SHOPPING LIST

- ☐ _____
- ☐ _____
- ☐ _____
- ☐ _____
- ☐ _____
- ☐ _____
- ☐ _____
- ☐ _____
- ☐ _____
- ☐ _____
- ☐ _____
- ☐ _____
- ☐ _____
- ☐ _____
- ☐ _____
- ☐ _____
- ☐ _____
- ☐ _____
- ☐ _____

"If you can dream it, you can do it."

WALT DISNEY

NOTES

SATURDAY	
B	
L	
D	

SUNDAY	
B	
L	
D	

Calories/Points Tracker

DATE ____ / ____ / ____ TO ____ / ____ / ____

	MONDAY		TUESDAY	
	FOODS	Calories/ Points	FOODS	Calories/ Points
BREAKFAST				
LUNCH				
DINNER				
SNACKS				
	DAILY TOTAL		DAILY TOTAL	

WEDNESDAY		THURSDAY	
FOODS	Calories/ Points	FOODS	Calories/ Points
DAILY TOTAL		DAILY TOTAL	

Calories/Points Tracker

DATE ___ / ___ / ___ TO ___ / ___ / ___

	FRIDAY			SATURDAY	
	FOODS	Calories/Points		FOODS	Calories/Points
BREAKFAST					
LUNCH					
DINNER					
SNACKS					
	DAILY TOTAL			DAILY TOTAL	

WEEKLY EXERCISE TRACKER

ACTIVITY	
DISTANCE/DURATION/INTENSITY	CALORIES BURNED

SUNDAY	
FOODS	Calories/Points
DAILY TOTAL	

TOTAL CALORIES BURNED	

MONDAY	-	=
TUESDAY	-	=
WEDNESDAY	-	=
THURSDAY	-	=
FRIDAY	-	=
SATURDAY	-	=
SUNDAY	-	=
WEEKLY CALORIES TOTALS	-	=
	Food	Exercise	Total

Weekly Meal Planner

DATE _____ / _____ / _____ TO _____ / _____ / _____

WEEKLY GOALS

1. _____

    M T W T F S S
    ☐ ☐ ☐ ☐ ☐ ☐ ☐

2. _____

    M T W T F S S
    ☐ ☐ ☐ ☐ ☐ ☐ ☐

3. _____

    M T W T F S S
    ☐ ☐ ☐ ☐ ☐ ☐ ☐

MONDAY

B

L

D

TUESDAY

B

L

D

WEDNESDAY

B

L

D

THURSDAY

B

L

D

FRIDAY

B

L

D

SHOPPING LIST

- [ ] _____
- [ ] _____
- [ ] _____
- [ ] _____
- [ ] _____
- [ ] _____
- [ ] _____
- [ ] _____
- [ ] _____
- [ ] _____
- [ ] _____
- [ ] _____
- [ ] _____
- [ ] _____
- [ ] _____
- [ ] _____
- [ ] _____
- [ ] _____
- [ ] _____

superfood FLAXSEEDS

There are two ways to eat flaxseeds: whole and mixed into things like granola and cereal, or ground and tossed into smoothies. Yum!

NOTES

	SATURDAY
B	
L	
D	

	SUNDAY
B	
L	
D	

Calories/Points Tracker

DATE _____ / _____ / _____ TO _____ / _____ / _____

	MONDAY			TUESDAY	
	FOODS	Calories/Points		FOODS	Calories/Points
BREAKFAST					
LUNCH					
DINNER					
SNACKS					
	DAILY TOTAL			DAILY TOTAL	

WEDNESDAY		THURSDAY	
FOODS	Calories/Points	FOODS	Calories/Points
DAILY TOTAL		DAILY TOTAL	

Calories/Points Tracker

DATE ___ / ___ / ___ TO ___ / ___ / ___

	FRIDAY			SATURDAY	
	FOODS	Calories/Points		FOODS	Calories/Points
BREAKFAST					
LUNCH					
DINNER					
SNACKS					
	DAILY TOTAL			DAILY TOTAL	

WEEKLY EXERCISE TRACKER

ACTIVITY	
DISTANCE/DURATION/INTENSITY	CALORIES BURNED

SUNDAY	
FOODS	Calories/ Points
DAILY TOTAL	

TOTAL CALORIES BURNED

MONDAY	-	=
TUESDAY	-	=
WEDNESDAY	-	=
THURSDAY	-	=
FRIDAY	-	=
SATURDAY	-	=
SUNDAY	-	=
WEEKLY CALORIES TOTALS	-	=
	Food	Exercise	Total

Weekly Meal Planner

DATE ____ / ____ / ____ TO ____ / ____ / ____

WEEKLY GOALS

1. _____ M T W T F S S
   □ □ □ □ □ □ □

2. _____ M T W T F S S
   □ □ □ □ □ □ □

3. _____ M T W T F S S
   □ □ □ □ □ □ □

MONDAY
B
L
D

TUESDAY
B
L
D

WEDNESDAY
B
L
D

THURSDAY
B
L
D

FRIDAY
B
L
D

SHOPPING LIST

- ☐ _____
- ☐ _____
- ☐ _____
- ☐ _____
- ☐ _____
- ☐ _____
- ☐ _____
- ☐ _____
- ☐ _____
- ☐ _____
- ☐ _____
- ☐ _____
- ☐ _____
- ☐ _____
- ☐ _____
- ☐ _____
- ☐ _____
- ☐ _____
- ☐ _____

> "The secret of getting ahead is getting started."
>
> MARK TWAIN

NOTES

_____
_____
_____
_____
_____
_____
_____
_____
_____
_____
_____

SATURDAY	
B	
L	
D	

SUNDAY	
B	
L	
D	

Calories/Points Tracker

DATE ___ / ___ / ___ TO ___ / ___ / ___

	MONDAY			TUESDAY	
	FOODS	Calories/Points		FOODS	Calories/Points
BREAKFAST					
LUNCH					
DINNER					
SNACKS					
	DAILY TOTAL			DAILY TOTAL	

WEDNESDAY		THURSDAY	
FOODS	Calories/Points	FOODS	Calories/Points
DAILY TOTAL		DAILY TOTAL	

Calories/Points Tracker

DATE _____ / _____ / _____ TO _____ / _____ / _____

	FRIDAY			SATURDAY	
	FOODS	Calories/Points		FOODS	Calories/Points
BREAKFAST					
LUNCH					
DINNER					
SNACKS					
	DAILY TOTAL			DAILY TOTAL	

WEEKLY EXERCISE TRACKER

SUNDAY	
FOODS	Calories/ Points
DAILY TOTAL	

ACTIVITY	
DISTANCE/DURATION/INTENSITY	CALORIES BURNED
TOTAL CALORIES BURNED	

MONDAY	-	=	
TUESDAY	-	=	
WEDNESDAY	-	=	
THURSDAY	-	=	
FRIDAY	-	=	
SATURDAY	-	=	
SUNDAY	-	=	
WEEKLY CALORIES TOTALS	-	=	
	Food	Exercise	Total

Weekly Meal Planner

DATE ____ / ____ / ____ TO ____ / ____ / ____

WEEKLY GOALS

1. _____   M T W T F S S
                                                        ☐ ☐ ☐ ☐ ☐ ☐ ☐

2. _____   M T W T F S S
                                                        ☐ ☐ ☐ ☐ ☐ ☐ ☐

3. _____   M T W T F S S
                                                        ☐ ☐ ☐ ☐ ☐ ☐ ☐

MONDAY	
B	
L	
D	

TUESDAY	
B	
L	
D	

WEDNESDAY	
B	
L	
D	

THURSDAY	
B	
L	
D	

FRIDAY	
B	
L	
D	

- ☐ _____
- ☐ _____
- ☐ _____
- ☐ _____
- ☐ _____
- ☐ _____
- ☐ _____
- ☐ _____
- ☐ _____
- ☐ _____
- ☐ _____
- ☐ _____
- ☐ _____
- ☐ _____
- ☐ _____
- ☐ _____
- ☐ _____
- ☐ _____
- ☐ _____
- ☐ _____

superfood

DARK CHOCOLATE

Here's your license to eat some chocolate! Just a small square a day will give your body a dose of healthy antioxidants.

NOTES

SATURDAY	
B	
L	
D	

SUNDAY	
B	
L	
D	

Calories/Points Tracker

DATE ___ / ___ / ___ TO ___ / ___ / ___

	MONDAY			TUESDAY	
	FOODS	Calories/ Points		FOODS	Calories/ Points
BREAKFAST					
LUNCH					
DINNER					
SNACKS					
	DAILY TOTAL			DAILY TOTAL	

WEDNESDAY		THURSDAY	
FOODS	Calories/ Points	FOODS	Calories/ Points
DAILY TOTAL		DAILY TOTAL	

Fettuccine with Winter Greens and Poached Egg

Pasta with greens and a poached egg is one of my favorite go-to, no-fuss weeknight dinners in the colder months when I'm hungry and need dinner on the table quick. I always have eggs, pasta, and some type of greens on hand, so the dish really does come together fast. The poached egg creates a luscious sauce when mixed into the pasta, and it is even better topped with freshly shaved Parmesan cheese.

SERVES 2

4 ounces dried egg fettuccine

2 large eggs

½ tablespoon olive oil

½ small red onion, thinly sliced

¼ teaspoon kosher salt

1 garlic clove, chopped

Leaves from 1 sprig of fresh thyme

4 ounces (4 cups) chopped winter greens, such as chard, escarole, spinach, or kale

Freshly shaved Parmesan, for serving (optional)

PER SERVING	1½ cups + 1 egg
CALORIES	322
FAT	10 g
SATURATED FAT	2.5 g
CHOLESTEROL	296 mg
CARBOHYDRATE	43 g
FIBER	3.5 g
PROTEIN	16 g
SUGAR	2 g
SODIUM	338 mg

In a medium pot of salted boiling water, cook the pasta to al dente according to the package directions. Drain, reserving 1 cup of the cooking water.

Meanwhile, to poach the eggs, in a large deep skillet, bring 1½ to 2 inches water to a boil over high heat. Reduce the heat to low to maintain a simmer. Crack the eggs into individual bowls. Gently slide the eggs into the simmering water one at a time. Using a spoon, gently nudge the egg whites toward the yolk. Cook for 2 to 3 minutes for a semisoft yolk, or 3 to 4 minutes for a firmer-set yolk. Using a slotted spoon or spatula, remove the eggs one at a time and drain on paper towels.

In a large skillet, combine the oil, red onion, and ⅛ teaspoon of the salt. Cook over medium-high heat, stirring occasionally, until the onion starts to caramelize, about 3 minutes. Stir in the garlic and thyme and cook until fragrant, about 1 minute. Add the greens and ¾ cup of the reserved cooking water. Bring to a boil, reduce the heat to low, and simmer until the greens turn bright green and are just tender, 2 to 3 minutes. Stir in the pasta and cook until heated through, 1 minute. Remove the pan from the heat and season with the remaining ⅛ teaspoon salt and pepper to taste.

Divide the pasta between 2 serving bowls. Top each with an egg, Parmesan (if using), and serve with more pepper, if desired. Serve.

Calories/Points Tracker

DATE ___ / ___ / ___ TO ___ / ___ / ___

	FRIDAY			SATURDAY	
	FOODS	Calories/Points		FOODS	Calories/Points
BREAKFAST					
LUNCH					
DINNER					
SNACKS					
	DAILY TOTAL			DAILY TOTAL	

WEEKLY EXERCISE TRACKER

SUNDAY	
FOODS	Calories/ Points
DAILY TOTAL	

ACTIVITY	
DISTANCE/DURATION/INTENSITY	CALORIES BURNED
TOTAL CALORIES BURNED	

MONDAY		-	=
TUESDAY		-	=
WEDNESDAY		-	=
THURSDAY		-	=
FRIDAY		-	=
SATURDAY		-	=
SUNDAY		-	=
WEEKLY CALORIES TOTALS	Food	Exercise	Total

Weekly Meal Planner

DATE ___ / ___ / ___ TO ___ / ___ / ___

WEEKLY GOALS

1. _____ M T W T F S S
   □ □ □ □ □ □ □

2. _____ M T W T F S S
   □ □ □ □ □ □ □

3. _____ M T W T F S S
   □ □ □ □ □ □ □

MONDAY	
B	
L	
D	

TUESDAY	
B	
L	
D	

WEDNESDAY	
B	
L	
D	

THURSDAY	
B	
L	
D	

FRIDAY	
B	
L	
D	

SHOPPING LIST

- [ ] _____
- [ ] _____
- [ ] _____
- [ ] _____
- [ ] _____
- [ ] _____
- [ ] _____
- [ ] _____
- [ ] _____
- [ ] _____
- [ ] _____
- [ ] _____
- [ ] _____
- [ ] _____
- [ ] _____
- [ ] _____
- [ ] _____
- [ ] _____
- [ ] _____

> "It's not the years in your life that count. It's the life in your years."
>
> ABRAHAM LINCOLN

NOTES

_____
_____
_____
_____
_____
_____
_____
_____
_____
_____
_____

SATURDAY	
B	
L	
D	

SUNDAY	
B	
L	
D	

Calories/Points Tracker

DATE ____ / ____ / ____ TO ____ / ____ / ____

	MONDAY			TUESDAY	
	FOODS	Calories/Points		FOODS	Calories/Points
BREAKFAST					
LUNCH					
DINNER					
SNACKS					
	DAILY TOTAL			DAILY TOTAL	

WEDNESDAY		THURSDAY	
FOODS	Calories/ Points	FOODS	Calories/ Points
DAILY TOTAL		DAILY TOTAL	

Calories/Points Tracker

DATE ___/___/___ TO ___/___/___

	FRIDAY			SATURDAY	
	FOODS	Calories/Points		FOODS	Calories/Points
BREAKFAST					
LUNCH					
DINNER					
SNACKS					
	DAILY TOTAL			DAILY TOTAL	

WEEKLY EXERCISE TRACKER

SUNDAY	
FOODS	Calories/ Points
DAILY TOTAL	

ACTIVITY		
DISTANCE/DURATION/INTENSITY		CALORIES BURNED
TOTAL CALORIES BURNED		

MONDAY		-	=
TUESDAY		-	=
WEDNESDAY		-	=
THURSDAY		-	=
FRIDAY		-	=
SATURDAY		-	=
SUNDAY		-	=
WEEKLY CALORIES TOTALS		-	=
	Food	Exercise	Total

Weekly Meal Planner

DATE _____ / ___ / _____ TO _____ / ___ / _____

WEEKLY GOALS

1. _____ M T W T F S S
   ☐ ☐ ☐ ☐ ☐ ☐ ☐

2. _____ M T W T F S S
   ☐ ☐ ☐ ☐ ☐ ☐ ☐

3. _____ M T W T F S S
   ☐ ☐ ☐ ☐ ☐ ☐ ☐

MONDAY	
B	
L	
D	

TUESDAY	
B	
L	
D	

WEDNESDAY	
B	
L	
D	

THURSDAY	
B	
L	
D	

FRIDAY	
B	
L	
D	

SHOPPING LIST

- [ ] _____
- [ ] _____
- [ ] _____
- [ ] _____
- [ ] _____
- [ ] _____
- [ ] _____
- [ ] _____
- [ ] _____
- [ ] _____
- [ ] _____
- [ ] _____
- [ ] _____
- [ ] _____
- [ ] _____
- [ ] _____
- [ ] _____
- [ ] _____
- [ ] _____

> "Change your thoughts and you change your world."
>
> NORMAN VINCENT PEALE

NOTES

_____
_____
_____
_____
_____
_____
_____
_____
_____
_____
_____
_____
_____
_____

SATURDAY	
B	
L	
D	

SUNDAY	
B	
L	
D	

Calories/Points Tracker

DATE ___ / ___ / ___ TO ___ / ___ / ___

	MONDAY			TUESDAY	
	FOODS	Calories/Points		FOODS	Calories/Points
BREAKFAST					
LUNCH					
DINNER					
SNACKS					
	DAILY TOTAL			DAILY TOTAL	

WEDNESDAY			THURSDAY	
FOODS	Calories/ Points		FOODS	Calories/ Points
DAILY TOTAL			DAILY TOTAL	

Calories/Points Tracker

DATE ___ / ___ / ___ TO ___ / ___ / ___

	FRIDAY			SATURDAY	
	FOODS	Calories/Points		FOODS	Calories/Points
BREAKFAST					
LUNCH					
DINNER					
SNACKS					
	DAILY TOTAL			DAILY TOTAL	

WEEKLY EXERCISE TRACKER

SUNDAY	
FOODS	Calories/ Points
DAILY TOTAL	

ACTIVITY		
DISTANCE/DURATION/INTENSITY		CALORIES BURNED
TOTAL CALORIES BURNED		

MONDAY	-	=	
TUESDAY	-	=	
WEDNESDAY	-	=	
THURSDAY	-	=	
FRIDAY	-	=	
SATURDAY	-	=	
SUNDAY	-	=	
WEEKLY CALORIES TOTALS	-	=	
	Food	Exercise	Total

Weekly Meal Planner

DATE ___ / ___ / ___ TO ___ / ___ / ___

WEEKLY GOALS

1. _____ M T W T F S S ☐☐☐☐☐☐☐

2. _____ M T W T F S S ☐☐☐☐☐☐☐

3. _____ M T W T F S S ☐☐☐☐☐☐☐

MONDAY	
B	
L	
D	

TUESDAY	
B	
L	
D	

WEDNESDAY	
B	
L	
D	

THURSDAY	
B	
L	
D	

FRIDAY	
B	
L	
D	

SHOPPING LIST

- [ ] _____
- [ ] _____
- [ ] _____
- [ ] _____
- [ ] _____
- [ ] _____
- [ ] _____
- [ ] _____
- [ ] _____
- [ ] _____
- [ ] _____
- [ ] _____
- [ ] _____
- [ ] _____
- [ ] _____
- [ ] _____
- [ ] _____
- [ ] _____
- [ ] _____

superfood GREEN TEA

Try swapping out a cup (or two) of coffee each day with green tea. You'll get the same caffeine pick-me-up, with more antioxidants for your body.

NOTES

_____
_____
_____
_____
_____
_____
_____
_____
_____
_____
_____

SATURDAY	
B	
L	
D	

SUNDAY	
B	
L	
D	

Calories/Points Tracker

DATE ___/___/___ TO ___/___/___

	MONDAY			TUESDAY	
	FOODS	Calories/Points		FOODS	Calories/Points
BREAKFAST					
LUNCH					
DINNER					
SNACKS					
	DAILY TOTAL			DAILY TOTAL	

WEDNESDAY		THURSDAY	
FOODS	Calories/ Points	FOODS	Calories/ Points
DAILY TOTAL		DAILY TOTAL	

Calories/Points Tracker

DATE ___ / ___ / ___ TO ___ / ___ / ___

	FRIDAY			SATURDAY	
	FOODS	Calories/Points		FOODS	Calories/Points
BREAKFAST					
LUNCH					
DINNER					
SNACKS					
	DAILY TOTAL			DAILY TOTAL	

WEEKLY EXERCISE TRACKER

SUNDAY	
FOODS	Calories/ Points
DAILY TOTAL	

ACTIVITY	
DISTANCE/DURATION/INTENSITY	CALORIES BURNED

TOTAL CALORIES BURNED

MONDAY	–	=	
TUESDAY	–	=	
WEDNESDAY	–	=	
THURSDAY	–	=	
FRIDAY	–	=	
SATURDAY	–	=	
SUNDAY	–	=	
WEEKLY CALORIES TOTALS	–	=	
	Food	Exercise	Total

Weekly Meal Planner

DATE ___/___/___ TO ___/___/___

WEEKLY GOALS

1. _____ M T W T F S S
   ☐ ☐ ☐ ☐ ☐ ☐ ☐

2. _____ M T W T F S S
   ☐ ☐ ☐ ☐ ☐ ☐ ☐

3. _____ M T W T F S S
   ☐ ☐ ☐ ☐ ☐ ☐ ☐

MONDAY	
B	
L	
D	

TUESDAY	
B	
L	
D	

WEDNESDAY	
B	
L	
D	

THURSDAY	
B	
L	
D	

FRIDAY	
B	
L	
D	

SHOPPING LIST

☐ _____
☐ _____
☐ _____
☐ _____
☐ _____
☐ _____
☐ _____
☐ _____
☐ _____
☐ _____
☐ _____
☐ _____
☐ _____
☐ _____
☐ _____
☐ _____
☐ _____
☐ _____
☐ _____
☐ _____

"Either I will find a way,
or I will make one."

PHILIP SIDNEY

NOTES

_____
_____
_____
_____
_____
_____
_____
_____
_____
_____
_____

SATURDAY	
B	
L	
D	

SUNDAY	
B	
L	
D	

Embarrassingly Easy Slow Cooker Salsa Chicken Thighs

This chicken could not be simpler, and, for a slow cooker dish, it's pretty quick! It's delicious served several ways: we've loved it in tacos, over a salad or rice, and as an enchilada filling.

SERVES 6

1½ pounds skinless chicken thighs, trimmed

1 teaspoon adobo seasoning (or salt)

1 cup chunky mild jarred salsa

¼ teaspoon garlic powder

¾ teaspoon ground cumin

Season the chicken with the adobo, put it in a slow cooker, and top with the salsa, garlic powder, and ½ teaspoon of the cumin.

Cover and cook on low for 4 hours. Transfer the chicken to a large plate and shred with two forks. Pour the liquid in the slow cooker into a bowl and set aside. Put the shredded chicken back into the slow cooker and stir in the remaining ¼ teaspoon cumin. Pour ¾ cup of the reserved liquid back into the slow cooker and cover until ready to serve.

PER SERVING	scant ½ cup
CALORIES	151
FAT	5 g
SATURATED FAT	1 g
CHOLESTEROL	107 mg
CARBOHYDRATE	3 g
FIBER	1 g
PROTEIN	23 g
SUGAR	0 g
SODIUM	536 mg

Slow Cooker Blissful Butternut Squash Soup

This is the easiest, creamiest, yummiest fall slow cooker soup recipe—perfect for all you butternut lovers out there! Using only 7 ingredients and very minimal prep, this dreamy squash soup will satisfy your soup-loving soul. It's also gluten-free and can be vegan. I sometimes like to garnish it with a drizzle of more coconut milk, chopped fresh chives, or pumpkin seeds.

SERVES 4

16 ounces (½ small) butternut squash, halved and seeded

16 ounces (½) buttercup or kabocha squash, halved and seeded

2 large shallots, quartered

2 cups reduced-sodium vegetable or chicken broth

¾ cup light coconut milk

Pinch of ground nutmeg

Freshly ground black pepper

PER SERVING	1¼ cups
CALORIES	152
FAT	2.5 g
SATURATED FAT	1.5 g
CHOLESTEROL	0 mg
CARBOHYDRATE	33 g
FIBER	8.5 g
PROTEIN	4 g
SUGAR	2 g
SODIUM	310 mg

Place the squash, shallots, and broth in a slow cooker. Cover and cook on high for 4 hours or on low for 8 hours, until the squash is soft and cooked through and a knife may be easily inserted into the flesh.

Remove the squash from the slow cooker and, when it is cool enough to handle, scoop the flesh from the skins and return the flesh to the slow cooker (discard the skins). Stir in the coconut milk, nutmeg, and black pepper to taste. Using an immersion blender, puree until smooth (or blend in batches in a stand blender). Serve hot.

Calories/Points Tracker

DATE ____ / ___ / ___ TO ____ / ___ / ___

	MONDAY			TUESDAY	
	FOODS	Calories/ Points		FOODS	Calories/ Points
BREAKFAST					
LUNCH					
DINNER					
SNACKS					
	DAILY TOTAL			DAILY TOTAL	

WEDNESDAY		THURSDAY	
FOODS	Calories/ Points	FOODS	Calories/ Points
DAILY TOTAL		DAILY TOTAL	

Calories/Points Tracker

DATE ___ / ___ / ___ TO ___ / ___ / ___

	FRIDAY			SATURDAY	
	FOODS	Calories/Points		FOODS	Calories/Points
BREAKFAST					
LUNCH					
DINNER					
SNACKS					
	DAILY TOTAL			DAILY TOTAL	

WEEKLY EXERCISE TRACKER

ACTIVITY	
DISTANCE/DURATION/INTENSITY	CALORIES BURNED

SUNDAY	
FOODS	Calories/Points
DAILY TOTAL	

TOTAL CALORIES BURNED	

MONDAY	-	=
TUESDAY	-	=
WEDNESDAY	-	=
THURSDAY	-	=
FRIDAY	-	=
SATURDAY	-	=
SUNDAY	-	=
WEEKLY CALORIES TOTALS	-	=
	Food	Exercise	Total

Weekly Meal Planner

DATE ____ / ____ / ____ TO ____ / ____ / ____

WEEKLY GOALS

1. _____ M T W T F S S ☐☐☐☐☐☐☐

2. _____ M T W T F S S ☐☐☐☐☐☐☐

3. _____ M T W T F S S ☐☐☐☐☐☐☐

MONDAY	
B	
L	
D	

TUESDAY	
B	
L	
D	

WEDNESDAY	
B	
L	
D	

THURSDAY	
B	
L	
D	

FRIDAY	
B	
L	
D	

SHOPPING LIST

- [ ] _____
- [ ] _____
- [ ] _____
- [ ] _____
- [ ] _____
- [ ] _____
- [ ] _____
- [ ] _____
- [ ] _____
- [ ] _____
- [ ] _____
- [ ] _____
- [ ] _____
- [ ] _____
- [ ] _____
- [ ] _____
- [ ] _____
- [ ] _____
- [ ] _____
- [ ] _____
- [ ] _____

superfood GARLIC

Though the taste may be strong to some, garlic is one of my favorite foods. I love its pungency in everything from a bright vinaigrette to roasted vegetables and meats.

NOTES

SATURDAY	
B	
L	
D	

SUNDAY	
B	
L	
D	

Calories/Points Tracker

DATE ___/___/___ TO ___/___/___

	MONDAY			TUESDAY	
	FOODS	Calories/ Points		FOODS	Calories/ Points
BREAKFAST					
LUNCH					
DINNER					
SNACKS					
	DAILY TOTAL			DAILY TOTAL	

WEDNESDAY		THURSDAY	
FOODS	Calories/Points	FOODS	Calories/Points
DAILY TOTAL		DAILY TOTAL	

Calories/Points Tracker

DATE ___ / ___ / ___ TO ___ / ___ / ___

	FRIDAY			SATURDAY	
	FOODS	Calories/Points		FOODS	Calories/Points
BREAKFAST					
LUNCH					
DINNER					
SNACKS					
	DAILY TOTAL			DAILY TOTAL	

DAILY CALORIES/ POINTS GOALS

WEEKLY EXERCISE TRACKER

SUNDAY	
FOODS	*Calories/ Points*
DAILY TOTAL	

ACTIVITY

DISTANCE/DURATION/INTENSITY	CALORIES BURNED

TOTAL CALORIES BURNED

MONDAY	−	=
TUESDAY	−	=
WEDNESDAY	−	=
THURSDAY	−	=
FRIDAY	−	=
SATURDAY	−	=
SUNDAY	−	=
WEEKLY CALORIES TOTALS	−	=
	Food	*Exercise*	*Total*

Weekly Meal Planner

DATE ___ / ___ / ___ TO ___ / ___ / ___

WEEKLY GOALS

1. _____ M T W T F S S
   □ □ □ □ □ □ □

2. _____ M T W T F S S
   □ □ □ □ □ □ □

3. _____ M T W T F S S
   □ □ □ □ □ □ □

MONDAY	
B	
L	
D	

TUESDAY	
B	
L	
D	

WEDNESDAY	
B	
L	
D	

THURSDAY	
B	
L	
D	

FRIDAY	
B	
L	
D	

SHOPPING LIST

- [ ] _____
- [ ] _____
- [ ] _____
- [ ] _____
- [ ] _____
- [ ] _____
- [ ] _____
- [ ] _____
- [ ] _____
- [ ] _____
- [ ] _____
- [ ] _____
- [ ] _____
- [ ] _____
- [ ] _____
- [ ] _____
- [ ] _____
- [ ] _____
- [ ] _____

> "If you ask me what I came into this life to do, I will tell you: I came to live out loud."
>
> ÉMILE ZOLA

NOTES

_____
_____
_____
_____
_____
_____
_____
_____
_____
_____
_____
_____

SATURDAY	
B	
L	
D	

SUNDAY	
B	
L	
D	

Calories/Points Tracker

DATE ___ / ___ / ___ TO ___ / ___ / ___

	MONDAY			TUESDAY	
	FOODS	Calories/Points		FOODS	Calories/Points
BREAKFAST					
LUNCH					
DINNER					
SNACKS					
	DAILY TOTAL			DAILY TOTAL	

WEDNESDAY			THURSDAY	
FOODS	Calories/Points		FOODS	Calories/Points
DAILY TOTAL			DAILY TOTAL	

Calories/Points Tracker

DATE ___ / ___ / ___ TO ___ / ___ / ___

	FRIDAY			SATURDAY	
	FOODS	Calories/Points		FOODS	Calories/Points
BREAKFAST					
LUNCH					
DINNER					
SNACKS					
	DAILY TOTAL			DAILY TOTAL	

WEEKLY EXERCISE TRACKER

SUNDAY	
FOODS	Calories/ Points
DAILY TOTAL	

ACTIVITY	
DISTANCE/DURATION/INTENSITY	CALORIES BURNED
TOTAL CALORIES BURNED	

MONDAY		-	=
TUESDAY		-	=
WEDNESDAY		-	=
THURSDAY		-	=
FRIDAY		-	=
SATURDAY		-	=
SUNDAY		-	=
WEEKLY CALORIES TOTALS		-	=
	Food	Exercise	Total

Weekly Meal Planner

DATE ___/___/___ TO ___/___/___

WEEKLY GOALS

1. _____ M T W T F S S
                                            ☐ ☐ ☐ ☐ ☐ ☐ ☐

2. _____ M T W T F S S
                                            ☐ ☐ ☐ ☐ ☐ ☐ ☐

3. _____ M T W T F S S
                                            ☐ ☐ ☐ ☐ ☐ ☐ ☐

MONDAY	
B	
L	
D	

TUESDAY	
B	
L	
D	

WEDNESDAY	
B	
L	
D	

THURSDAY	
B	
L	
D	

FRIDAY	
B	
L	
D	

- [ ] _____
- [ ] _____
- [ ] _____
- [ ] _____
- [ ] _____
- [ ] _____
- [ ] _____
- [ ] _____
- [ ] _____
- [ ] _____
- [ ] _____
- [ ] _____
- [ ] _____
- [ ] _____
- [ ] _____
- [ ] _____
- [ ] _____
- [ ] _____
- [ ] _____

"Be in love with your
life. Every minute of it."

JACK KEROUAC

NOTES

SATURDAY	
B	
L	
D	

SUNDAY	
B	
L	
D	

Calories/Points Tracker

DATE ____ / ____ / ____ TO ____ / ____ / ____

	MONDAY			TUESDAY	
	FOODS	Calories/ Points		FOODS	Calories/ Points
BREAKFAST					
LUNCH					
DINNER					
SNACKS					
	DAILY TOTAL			DAILY TOTAL	

WEDNESDAY		THURSDAY	
FOODS	Calories/ Points	FOODS	Calories/ Points
DAILY TOTAL		DAILY TOTAL	

Calories/Points Tracker

	FRIDAY		SATURDAY	
	FOODS	Calories/Points	FOODS	Calories/Points
BREAKFAST				
LUNCH				
DINNER				
SNACKS				
	DAILY TOTAL		DAILY TOTAL	

WEEKLY EXERCISE TRACKER

ACTIVITY	
DISTANCE/DURATION/INTENSITY	CALORIES BURNED

SUNDAY	
FOODS	Calories/ Points
DAILY TOTAL	

TOTAL CALORIES BURNED	

MONDAY	–	=	
TUESDAY	–	=	
WEDNESDAY	–	=	
THURSDAY	–	=	
FRIDAY	–	=	
SATURDAY	–	=	
SUNDAY	–	=	
WEEKLY CALORIES TOTALS	–	=	
	Food	Exercise	Total

Grilled Chicken Salad
with Strawberries and Spinach

I adore strawberries and could eat this salad all summer long when the berries are at their peak. Here I've made it with creamy goat cheese and a golden balsamic dressing, but it would also be great with feta cheese. If you want to add more protein, or to skip the cheese, add walnuts or slivered almonds.

SERVES 4

DRESSING

- 3 tablespoons extra-virgin olive oil
- 3 tablespoons golden balsamic vinegar
- 1 teaspoon honey
- 1 tablespoon chopped shallot
- ⅛ teaspoon kosher salt
- Freshly ground black pepper

CHICKEN

- 1 pound boneless, skinless chicken breasts
- 1 teaspoon seasoned salt (I like Grill Mates Montreal Steak seasoning)
- 1 garlic clove, crushed with the side of a knife
- Olive oil or olive oil spray, for greasing

SALAD

- 6 cups baby spinach
- 3 cups sliced strawberries
- 2 ounces soft goat cheese

PER SERVING	1½ cups salad + 3 ounces chicken
CALORIES	331
FAT	17 g
SATURATED FAT	4 g
CHOLESTEROL	90 mg
CARBOHYDRATE	15 g
FIBER	4 g
PROTEIN	31 g
SUGAR	11 g
SODIUM	347 mg

FOR THE DRESSING: In a small bowl, whisk together the oil, vinegar, honey, 1 teaspoon water, the shallot, salt, and pepper to taste.

FOR THE CHICKEN: Sprinkle the chicken all over with the seasoned salt, then rub on the crushed garlic.

Preheat a grill to medium (or preheat a grill pan over medium heat). Lightly rub the grates with oil (or spray the grill pan with olive oil). Grill the chicken on each side until charred on the outside and cooked through, 10 to 11 minutes total. Transfer to a cutting board and slice on an angle.

FOR THE SALAD: In a large bowl, toss the spinach with the dressing. Divide among 4 plates and top with the strawberries, goat cheese, and grilled chicken. Serve.

Weekly Meal Planner

DATE ___ / ___ / ___ TO ___ / ___ / ___

WEEKLY GOALS

1. _____ M T W T F S S
                                                     ☐ ☐ ☐ ☐ ☐ ☐ ☐

2. _____ M T W T F S S
                                                     ☐ ☐ ☐ ☐ ☐ ☐ ☐

3. _____ M T W T F S S
                                                     ☐ ☐ ☐ ☐ ☐ ☐ ☐

MONDAY
B
L
D

TUESDAY
B
L
D

WEDNESDAY
B
L
D

THURSDAY
B
L
D

FRIDAY
B
L
D

SHOPPING LIST

- [ ] _____
- [ ] _____
- [ ] _____
- [ ] _____
- [ ] _____
- [ ] _____
- [ ] _____
- [ ] _____
- [ ] _____
- [ ] _____
- [ ] _____
- [ ] _____
- [ ] _____
- [ ] _____
- [ ] _____
- [ ] _____
- [ ] _____
- [ ] _____
- [ ] _____

superfood OLIVE OIL

This healthy oil should always be at hand in your kitchen! Use it wherever possible in place of other oils or butter.

NOTES

_____
_____
_____
_____
_____
_____
_____
_____
_____
_____
_____

SATURDAY	
B	
L	
D	

SUNDAY	
B	
L	
D	

Calories/Points Tracker

	MONDAY			TUESDAY	
	FOODS	Calories/ Points		FOODS	Calories/ Points
BREAKFAST					
LUNCH					
DINNER					
SNACKS					
	DAILY TOTAL			DAILY TOTAL	

WEDNESDAY		THURSDAY	
FOODS	Calories/ Points	FOODS	Calories/ Points
DAILY TOTAL		DAILY TOTAL	

Calories/Points Tracker

DATE ___ / ___ / ___ TO ___ / ___ / ___

	FRIDAY			SATURDAY	
	FOODS	Calories/ Points		FOODS	Calories/ Points
BREAKFAST					
LUNCH					
DINNER					
SNACKS					
	DAILY TOTAL			DAILY TOTAL	

DAILY CALORIES/ POINTS GOALS

WEEKLY EXERCISE TRACKER

SUNDAY	
FOODS	Calories/ Points
DAILY TOTAL	

ACTIVITY	
DISTANCE/DURATION/INTENSITY	CALORIES BURNED
TOTAL CALORIES BURNED	

MONDAY		-	=
TUESDAY		-	=
WEDNESDAY		-	=
THURSDAY		-	=
FRIDAY		-	=
SATURDAY		-	=
SUNDAY		-	=
WEEKLY CALORIES TOTALS		-	=
	Food	Exercise	Total

Weekly Meal Planner

DATE ____ / ____ / ____ TO ____ / ____ / ____

WEEKLY GOALS

1. _____ M T W T F S S
   ☐ ☐ ☐ ☐ ☐ ☐ ☐

2. _____ M T W T F S S
   ☐ ☐ ☐ ☐ ☐ ☐ ☐

3. _____ M T W T F S S
   ☐ ☐ ☐ ☐ ☐ ☐ ☐

MONDAY	
B	
L	
D	

TUESDAY	
B	
L	
D	

WEDNESDAY	
B	
L	
D	

THURSDAY	
B	
L	
D	

FRIDAY	
B	
L	
D	

SHOPPING LIST

- [ ] _____
- [ ] _____
- [ ] _____
- [ ] _____
- [ ] _____
- [ ] _____
- [ ] _____
- [ ] _____
- [ ] _____
- [ ] _____
- [ ] _____
- [ ] _____
- [ ] _____
- [ ] _____
- [ ] _____
- [ ] _____
- [ ] _____
- [ ] _____
- [ ] _____

> "There are two ways of spreading light: to be the candle or the mirror that reflects it."
>
> EDITH WHARTON

NOTES

_____
_____
_____
_____
_____
_____
_____
_____
_____
_____
_____
_____
_____

SATURDAY	
B	
L	
D	

SUNDAY	
B	
L	
D	

Calories/Points Tracker

DATE ____ / ____ / ____ TO ____ / ____ / ____

	MONDAY			TUESDAY	
	FOODS	Calories/Points		FOODS	Calories/Points
BREAKFAST					
LUNCH					
DINNER					
SNACKS					
	DAILY TOTAL			DAILY TOTAL	

WEDNESDAY			THURSDAY	
FOODS	Calories/ Points		FOODS	Calories/ Points
DAILY TOTAL			DAILY TOTAL	

Calories/Points Tracker

DATE ___ / ___ / ___ TO ___ / ___ / ___

	FRIDAY			SATURDAY	
	FOODS	Calories/Points		FOODS	Calories/Points
BREAKFAST					
LUNCH					
DINNER					
SNACKS					
	DAILY TOTAL			DAILY TOTAL	

WEEKLY EXERCISE TRACKER

ACTIVITY	
DISTANCE/DURATION/INTENSITY	CALORIES BURNED

SUNDAY	
FOODS	Calories/ Points
DAILY TOTAL	

TOTAL CALORIES BURNED

MONDAY	-	=
TUESDAY	-	=
WEDNESDAY	-	=
THURSDAY	-	=
FRIDAY	-	=
SATURDAY	-	=
SUNDAY	-	=
WEEKLY CALORIES TOTALS	-	=
	Food	Exercise	Total

Weekly Meal Planner

DATE ___/___/___ TO ___/___/___

WEEKLY GOALS

1. _____   M T W T F S S
                                                        ☐ ☐ ☐ ☐ ☐ ☐ ☐

2. _____   M T W T F S S
                                                        ☐ ☐ ☐ ☐ ☐ ☐ ☐

3. _____   M T W T F S S
                                                        ☐ ☐ ☐ ☐ ☐ ☐ ☐

MONDAY
B
L
D

TUESDAY
B
L
D

WEDNESDAY
B
L
D

THURSDAY
B
L
D

FRIDAY
B
L
D

SHOPPING LIST

- [ ] _____
- [ ] _____
- [ ] _____
- [ ] _____
- [ ] _____
- [ ] _____
- [ ] _____
- [ ] _____
- [ ] _____
- [ ] _____
- [ ] _____
- [ ] _____
- [ ] _____
- [ ] _____
- [ ] _____
- [ ] _____
- [ ] _____
- [ ] _____
- [ ] _____

superfood AVOCADOS

With a subtle flavor and creamy texture, avocados are really versatile. Try avocado toast: toasted bread topped with mashed avocado and sea salt.

NOTES

_____
_____
_____
_____
_____
_____
_____
_____
_____
_____
_____

SATURDAY	
B	
L	
D	

SUNDAY	
B	
L	
D	

Calories/Points Tracker

DATE ___ / ___ / ___ TO ___ / ___ / ___

	MONDAY			TUESDAY	
	FOODS	Calories/Points		FOODS	Calories/Points
BREAKFAST					
BREAKFAST					
BREAKFAST					
BREAKFAST					
BREAKFAST					
BREAKFAST					
BREAKFAST					
LUNCH					
LUNCH					
LUNCH					
LUNCH					
LUNCH					
LUNCH					
LUNCH					
DINNER					
DINNER					
DINNER					
DINNER					
DINNER					
DINNER					
DINNER					
SNACKS					
SNACKS					
	DAILY TOTAL			DAILY TOTAL	

WEDNESDAY		THURSDAY	
FOODS	Calories/ Points	FOODS	Calories/ Points
DAILY TOTAL		DAILY TOTAL	

Calories/Points Tracker

DATE ___ / ___ / ___ TO ___ / ___ / ___

	FRIDAY			SATURDAY	
	FOODS	Calories/Points		FOODS	Calories/Points
BREAKFAST					
LUNCH					
DINNER					
SNACKS					
	DAILY TOTAL			DAILY TOTAL	

WEEKLY EXERCISE TRACKER

ACTIVITY		
DISTANCE/DURATION/INTENSITY		CALORIES BURNED

SUNDAY	
FOODS	Calories/ Points
DAILY TOTAL	

TOTAL CALORIES BURNED	

MONDAY	-	=	
TUESDAY	-	=	
WEDNESDAY	-	=	
THURSDAY	-	=	
FRIDAY	-	=	
SATURDAY	-	=	
SUNDAY	-	=	
WEEKLY CALORIES TOTALS	-	=	
	Food	Exercise	Total

Weekly Meal Planner

DATE ___ / ___ / ___ TO ___ / ___ / ___

WEEKLY GOALS

1. _____ M T W T F S S
   ☐ ☐ ☐ ☐ ☐ ☐ ☐

2. _____ M T W T F S S
   ☐ ☐ ☐ ☐ ☐ ☐ ☐

3. _____ M T W T F S S
   ☐ ☐ ☐ ☐ ☐ ☐ ☐

MONDAY	
B	
L	
D	

TUESDAY	
B	
L	
D	

WEDNESDAY	
B	
L	
D	

THURSDAY	
B	
L	
D	

FRIDAY	
B	
L	
D	

SHOPPING LIST

- [ ] _____
- [ ] _____
- [ ] _____
- [ ] _____
- [ ] _____
- [ ] _____
- [ ] _____
- [ ] _____
- [ ] _____
- [ ] _____
- [ ] _____
- [ ] _____
- [ ] _____
- [ ] _____
- [ ] _____
- [ ] _____
- [ ] _____
- [ ] _____
- [ ] _____

> "Once you choose hope, anything's possible."
>
> CHRISTOPHER REEVE

NOTES

_____
_____
_____
_____
_____
_____
_____
_____
_____
_____
_____
_____
_____

SATURDAY	
B	
L	
D	

SUNDAY	
B	
L	
D	

Calories/Points Tracker

DATE _____ / _____ / _____ TO _____ / _____ / _____

	MONDAY			TUESDAY	
	FOODS	Calories/Points		FOODS	Calories/Points
BREAKFAST					
LUNCH					
DINNER					
SNACKS					
	DAILY TOTAL			DAILY TOTAL	

WEDNESDAY			THURSDAY	
FOODS	Calories/ Points		FOODS	Calories/ Points
DAILY TOTAL			DAILY TOTAL	

Grilled Shrimp Salad with Orange, Endive, Arugula, and Radicchio

Once the weather begins warming up, I start eating lots of salads! This one is so tasty—my husband loves it, too—and it takes less than 15 minutes to make. I use my grill pan, but you can also put the shrimp on skewers and grill them outdoors. This dish is great warm or chilled, so you can definitely make the shrimp ahead.

SERVES 4

1 pound peeled and deveined jumbo shrimp

½ teaspoon kosher salt

4 teaspoons extra-virgin olive oil

Juice of 1 lemon

1 garlic clove, crushed with the side of a knife

Olive oil spray or olive oil, for greasing

1 cup arugula

3 Belgian endives, chopped

1 cup torn radicchio

1 navel orange, peeled, sectioned, and removed from the membrane

Juice of 1 navel orange

Freshly ground black pepper

PER SERVING	1½ cups
CALORIES	254
FAT	7.5 g
SATURATED FAT	1 g
CHOLESTEROL	172 mg
CARBOHYDRATE	21 g
FIBER	13 g
PROTEIN	29 g
SUGAR	6 g
SODIUM	396 mg

In a large bowl, season the shrimp with ¼ teaspoon of the salt. Add 1 teaspoon of the oil, half of the lemon juice, and the garlic and toss well.

Preheat a grill pan over medium-high heat (or preheat a grill to medium-high). When hot, spray the pan with olive oil (or rub the grill grates with oil). Cook the shrimp until just cooked through and opaque, about 2 minutes per side. Transfer to a large bowl and let cool. If you aren't making the salad right away, store the shrimp in an airtight container in the refrigerator for up to 2 days.

Into the bowl of shrimp, toss the arugula, endives, radicchio, orange sections, orange juice, remaining lemon juice, remaining 3 teaspoons oil, remaining ¼ teaspoon salt, and pepper to taste. Serve hot.

Calories/Points Tracker

DATE ___ / ___ / ___ TO ___ / ___ / ___

	FRIDAY		SATURDAY	
	FOODS	Calories/Points	FOODS	Calories/Points
BREAKFAST				
LUNCH				
DINNER				
SNACKS				
	DAILY TOTAL		DAILY TOTAL	

WEEKLY EXERCISE TRACKER

SUNDAY	
FOODS	Calories/ Points
DAILY TOTAL	

ACTIVITY	
DISTANCE/DURATION/INTENSITY	CALORIES BURNED
TOTAL CALORIES BURNED	

MONDAY	–	=	
TUESDAY	–	=	
WEDNESDAY	–	=	
THURSDAY	–	=	
FRIDAY	–	=	
SATURDAY	–	=	
SUNDAY	–	=	
WEEKLY CALORIES TOTALS	–	=	
	Food	Exercise	Total

Weekly Meal Planner

DATE ___ / ___ / ___ TO ___ / ___ / ___

WEEKLY GOALS

1. _____ M T W T F S S
☐ ☐ ☐ ☐ ☐ ☐ ☐

2. _____ M T W T F S S
☐ ☐ ☐ ☐ ☐ ☐ ☐

3. _____ M T W T F S S
☐ ☐ ☐ ☐ ☐ ☐ ☐

MONDAY	
B	
L	
D	

TUESDAY	
B	
L	
D	

WEDNESDAY	
B	
L	
D	

THURSDAY	
B	
L	
D	

FRIDAY	
B	
L	
D	

SHOPPING LIST

- [ ] _____
- [ ] _____
- [ ] _____
- [ ] _____
- [ ] _____
- [ ] _____
- [ ] _____
- [ ] _____
- [ ] _____
- [ ] _____
- [ ] _____
- [ ] _____
- [ ] _____
- [ ] _____
- [ ] _____
- [ ] _____
- [ ] _____
- [ ] _____
- [ ] _____

"Every moment is a
fresh beginning."

T. S. ELIOT

NOTES

	SATURDAY
B	
L	
D	

	SUNDAY
B	
L	
D	

Calories/Points Tracker

DATE ___ / ___ / ___ TO ___ / ___ / ___

	MONDAY			TUESDAY	
	FOODS	Calories/ Points		FOODS	Calories/ Points
BREAKFAST					
LUNCH					
DINNER					
SNACKS					
	DAILY TOTAL			DAILY TOTAL	

WEDNESDAY		THURSDAY	
FOODS	Calories/Points	FOODS	Calories/Points
DAILY TOTAL		DAILY TOTAL	

Calories/Points Tracker

DATE ___ / ___ / ___ TO ___ / ___ / ___

	FRIDAY			SATURDAY	
	FOODS	Calories/ Points		FOODS	Calories/ Points
BREAKFAST					
LUNCH					
DINNER					
SNACKS					
	DAILY TOTAL			DAILY TOTAL	

WEEKLY EXERCISE TRACKER

SUNDAY	
FOODS	*Calories/ Points*
DAILY TOTAL	

ACTIVITY	
DISTANCE/DURATION/INTENSITY	CALORIES BURNED
TOTAL CALORIES BURNED	

	Food	Exercise	Total
MONDAY	−	=	
TUESDAY	−	=	
WEDNESDAY	−	=	
THURSDAY	−	=	
FRIDAY	−	=	
SATURDAY	−	=	
SUNDAY	−	=	
WEEKLY CALORIES TOTALS	−	=	

Weekly Meal Planner

DATE ____ / ____ / ____ TO ____ / ____ / ____

WEEKLY GOALS

1. _____ M T W T F S S
   ◻ ◻ ◻ ◻ ◻ ◻ ◻

2. _____ M T W T F S S
   ◻ ◻ ◻ ◻ ◻ ◻ ◻

3. _____ M T W T F S S
   ◻ ◻ ◻ ◻ ◻ ◻ ◻

MONDAY
B
L
D

TUESDAY
B
L
D

WEDNESDAY
B
L
D

THURSDAY
B
L
D

FRIDAY
B
L
D

SHOPPING LIST

- [ ] _____
- [ ] _____
- [ ] _____
- [ ] _____
- [ ] _____
- [ ] _____
- [ ] _____
- [ ] _____
- [ ] _____
- [ ] _____
- [ ] _____
- [ ] _____
- [ ] _____
- [ ] _____
- [ ] _____
- [ ] _____
- [ ] _____
- [ ] _____

superfood TOMATOES

Take advantage of those gorgeous summer tomatoes! Slice heirloom varieties for a stunning salad, and make a weekend project out of canning fresh sauce. You'll be thankful come winter!

NOTES

_____
_____
_____
_____
_____
_____
_____
_____
_____

SATURDAY	
B	
L	
D	

SUNDAY	
B	
L	
D	

Calories/Points Tracker

DATE ___ / ___ / ___ TO ___ / ___ / ___

	MONDAY			TUESDAY	
	FOODS	Calories/ Points		FOODS	Calories/ Points
BREAKFAST					
LUNCH					
DINNER					
SNACKS					
	DAILY TOTAL			DAILY TOTAL	

WEDNESDAY		THURSDAY	
FOODS	Calories/ Points	FOODS	Calories/ Points
DAILY TOTAL		DAILY TOTAL	

Calories/Points Tracker

DATE ____/____/____ TO ____/____/____

	FRIDAY			SATURDAY	
	FOODS	Calories/ Points		FOODS	Calories/ Points
BREAKFAST					
LUNCH					
DINNER					
SNACKS					
	DAILY TOTAL			DAILY TOTAL	

SUNDAY	
FOODS	Calories/ Points
DAILY TOTAL	

WEEKLY EXERCISE TRACKER

ACTIVITY	
DISTANCE/DURATION/INTENSITY	CALORIES BURNED
TOTAL CALORIES BURNED	

MONDAY	−	=	
TUESDAY	−	=	
WEDNESDAY	−	=	
THURSDAY	−	=	
FRIDAY	−	=	
SATURDAY	−	=	
SUNDAY	−	=	
WEEKLY CALORIES TOTALS	−	=	
	Food	Exercise	Total

Weekly Meal Planner

DATE ___ / ___ / ___ TO ___ / ___ / ___

WEEKLY GOALS

M T W T F S S
1. _____ ☐☐☐☐☐☐☐

M T W T F S S
2. _____ ☐☐☐☐☐☐☐

M T W T F S S
3. _____ ☐☐☐☐☐☐☐

MONDAY	
B	
L	
D	

TUESDAY	
B	
L	
D	

WEDNESDAY	
B	
L	
D	

THURSDAY	
B	
L	
D	

FRIDAY	
B	
L	
D	

SHOPPING LIST

- [ ] _____
- [ ] _____
- [ ] _____
- [ ] _____
- [ ] _____
- [ ] _____
- [ ] _____
- [ ] _____
- [ ] _____
- [ ] _____
- [ ] _____
- [ ] _____
- [ ] _____
- [ ] _____
- [ ] _____
- [ ] _____
- [ ] _____
- [ ] _____
- [ ] _____

> "Don't count the days,
> make the days count."
>
> MUHAMMAD ALI

NOTES

_____
_____
_____
_____
_____
_____
_____
_____
_____
_____
_____

SATURDAY	
B	
L	
D	

SUNDAY	
B	
L	
D	

Calories/Points Tracker

DATE ___ / ___ / ___ TO ___ / ___ / ___

	MONDAY			TUESDAY	
	FOODS	Calories/Points		FOODS	Calories/Points
BREAKFAST					
LUNCH					
DINNER					
SNACKS					
	DAILY TOTAL			DAILY TOTAL	

WEDNESDAY		THURSDAY	
FOODS	Calories/ Points	FOODS	Calories/ Points
DAILY TOTAL		DAILY TOTAL	

Calories/Points Tracker

DATE ___/___/___ TO ___/___/___

	FRIDAY			SATURDAY	
	FOODS	Calories/Points		FOODS	Calories/Points
BREAKFAST					
LUNCH					
DINNER					
SNACKS					
	DAILY TOTAL			DAILY TOTAL	

WEEKLY EXERCISE TRACKER

SUNDAY	
FOODS	Calories/ Points
DAILY TOTAL	

ACTIVITY	
DISTANCE/DURATION/INTENSITY	CALORIES BURNED

TOTAL CALORIES BURNED

MONDAY	-	=	
TUESDAY	-	=	
WEDNESDAY	-	=	
THURSDAY	-	=	
FRIDAY	-	=	
SATURDAY	-	=	
SUNDAY	-	=	
WEEKLY CALORIES TOTALS	-	=	
	Food	Exercise	Total

Weekly Meal Planner

DATE ____ / ____ / ____ TO ____ / ____ / ____

WEEKLY GOALS

1. _____ M T W T F S S ☐☐☐☐☐☐☐

2. _____ M T W T F S S ☐☐☐☐☐☐☐

3. _____ M T W T F S S ☐☐☐☐☐☐☐

MONDAY	
B	
L	
D	

TUESDAY	
B	
L	
D	

WEDNESDAY	
B	
L	
D	

THURSDAY	
B	
L	
D	

FRIDAY	
B	
L	
D	

SHOPPING LIST

☐ _____
☐ _____
☐ _____
☐ _____
☐ _____
☐ _____
☐ _____
☐ _____
☐ _____
☐ _____
☐ _____
☐ _____
☐ _____
☐ _____
☐ _____
☐ _____
☐ _____
☐ _____
☐ _____

"It always seems impossible until it's done."

NELSON MANDELA

NOTES

_____
_____
_____
_____
_____
_____
_____
_____
_____
_____
_____
_____

SATURDAY	
B	
L	
D	

SUNDAY	
B	
L	
D	

Sheet-Pan Shrimp with Broccolini and Tomatoes

One of my favorite ways to cook shrimp is to roast it in the oven—it comes out tender and flavorful every time. Once, I added some of our favorite vegetables to make a one-pan meal, and we loved it. A quick and easy low-carb dish with tons of flavor, this dinner is ready in under 30 minutes start to finish.

SERVES 4

- 1 pound (28 count) extra-large peeled, deveined, tail-off shrimp
- 2 tablespoons plus 2 teaspoons extra-virgin olive oil
- 3 garlic cloves, minced
- ¾ teaspoon kosher salt
- ⅛ teaspoon crushed red pepper flakes (optional)
- Freshly ground black pepper
- Olive oil spray
- 2 bunches (12 ounces total) broccolini (12 spears total), ends trimmed
- 1 cup grape tomatoes, halved
- 1 teaspoon chopped fresh oregano
- 2 tablespoons fresh lemon juice

PER SERVING	7 shrimp + 3 spears broccolini + tomatoes
CALORIES	238
FAT	12 g
SATURATED FAT	1.5 g
CHOLESTEROL	172 mg
CARBOHYDRATE	9 g
FIBER	3 g
PROTEIN	26 g
SUGAR	0 g
SODIUM	405 mg

Preheat the oven to 400°F.

In a medium bowl, toss together the shrimp, 2 teaspoons of the olive oil, the garlic, ¼ teaspoon of the salt, the pepper flakes (if using), and black pepper to taste.

Spray a large rimmed baking sheet with olive oil. Put the broccolini and tomatoes on the baking sheet and toss with the remaining 2 tablespoons olive oil, remaining ½ teaspoon salt, the oregano, and black pepper to taste. Spread the vegetables out in an even layer.

Roast for 15 minutes, tossing halfway through. Remove the baking sheet from the oven and add the shrimp, placing them evenly around the veggies. Roast until the shrimp are opaque, about 8 minutes. Sprinkle the lemon juice over everything and serve.

Calories/Points Tracker

DATE ___ / ___ / ___ TO ___ / ___ / ___

	MONDAY				TUESDAY		
	FOODS	Calories/Points			FOODS	Calories/Points	
BREAKFAST							
LUNCH							
DINNER							
SNACKS							
	DAILY TOTAL				DAILY TOTAL		

WEDNESDAY		THURSDAY	
FOODS	Calories/ Points	FOODS	Calories/ Points
DAILY TOTAL		DAILY TOTAL	

Calories/Points Tracker

DATE _____ / _____ / _____ TO _____ / _____ / _____

	FRIDAY			SATURDAY	
	FOODS	Calories/Points		FOODS	Calories/Points
BREAKFAST					
LUNCH					
DINNER					
SNACKS					
	DAILY TOTAL			DAILY TOTAL	

WEEKLY EXERCISE TRACKER

SUNDAY	
FOODS	Calories/ Points
DAILY TOTAL	

ACTIVITY	
DISTANCE/DURATION/INTENSITY	CALORIES BURNED
TOTAL CALORIES BURNED	

MONDAY	−	=
TUESDAY	−	=
WEDNESDAY	−	=
THURSDAY	−	=
FRIDAY	−	=
SATURDAY	−	=
SUNDAY	−	=
WEEKLY CALORIES TOTALS	−	=
	Food	Exercise	Total

POTTER

Copyright © 2015, 2017 by Gina Homolka
Illustrations copyright © 2015 by Shutterstock

All rights reserved.

Published in the United States by Clarkson Potter/Publishers,
an imprint of the Crown Publishing Group, a division
of Penguin Random House LLC, New York.

crownpublishing.com
clarksonpotter.com

CLARKSON POTTER is a trademark and POTTER with
colophon is a registered trademark of Penguin Random House LLC.

Skinnytaste™ is a trademark of Skinnytaste, Inc.

ISBN 978-0-525-57336-4
Printed in China

Illustrations by Shutterstock © Shizayats (carrot);
Texturis (all other vegetables and herb pattern)

10 9 8 7 6 5 4

Revised Edition